NO EGO
NO STRESS

Tao Wisdom
for
Stress Relief

STEPHEN LAU

All the quotes from Lao Tzu are taken from the author's own book:
The Complete TAO TE CHING in Plain English.

CONTENTS

THE AUTHOR'S NOTE

This book contains the whole script of the 81 chapters of **Lao Tzu**'s immortal classic **TAO TE CHING**, which underlies his wisdom (known as the TAO). Understanding his profound wisdom may help you let go of your ego-self, which is not only the source of all human miseries but also the underlying cause of human stress and sorrow.

Live your life free from stress and live it as if everything is a miracle. In order to do just that, you need to let go of your ego, which requires wisdom, more specifically, the wisdom of Lao Tzu, the ancient sage from China thousands of years ago.

The TAO focuses on the need of "emptying" and "reversing" the human mind in order to see "who" and "what" you truly are, without any attachment to the material world to define your identity or to inflate your ego-self, which is only your false identity.

According to Lao Tzu, the ego is unreal, because it is based on your past memories and projections of those memories into the future as your desires and expectations. The past is gone, the future is yet to come, and only the present is real. Therefore, the ego-self in the past or in the future is non-existing in the present, except in the mind. Without the ego, there is no need of protecting or sustaining it. Without fear and expectation, there is no need of judging, picking and choosing—they often result in making wrong choices and decisions, and thus creating stress. With no ego, there is no need of over-doing to fulfill all the expectations.

The problem with the conventional wisdom is that the mind focuses too much on the past or the future, but seldom stays in the present. Only when the mind stays in the present can it see things as they really are and not as what they should be.

The TAO is essentially the profound understanding of the true nature of all things: that everything in life follows a natural order and pattern, such as life begets death, success is followed by failure, and what goes up must also come down. The TAO is your self-intuition to know your true self, as well as to understand others and the world around you.

Stephen Lau

ONE

THE INTRODUCTION TO STRESS

Stress, Distress, and Chronic Stress

Stress is your body's response to increased tension. Stress is natural and normal. You need stress to do many things in life, such as accepting challenges, concentrating on doing a difficult task, and making important daily and life decisions, among others. Indeed, stress can be conducive to your health, such as stress from having sex, which increases both your pulse rate and heartbeat, as well as stimulates your brain cells to keep your brain younger and healthier for longer. In many ways, stress can be enjoyable, such as the mental and physical challenge in competitive games and sports.

After the initial stress-induced stimuli, your body should be able to relax, slow down, and then return to its original state of balance and equilibrium. If that does not happen, you may become distressed or even over-stressed. Too much stress can also increase your production of hormone epinephrine, and thus wearing out your hormonal glands. Dysfunctional hormone production may lead to many health issues: your blood sugar elevation to produce more energy; your breathing rate acceleration to get more oxygen to your lungs; your muscle tension; your pulse rate and blood pressure increase; and your excess sweating to cool down your body, among many other health issues. Yes, stress can be damaging to your overall health.

Staying slightly stressed every now and then is okay, but avoid distress—which is alienation, anxiety, fear, frustration, and even depression. When stress continues over long periods of time, it may become chronic stress, which is harmful and damaging to the body, the mind, and the soul.

The Damage and Devastation of Stress

Chronic stress, which causes the body to maintain physiological reactions for long periods of time, especially with respect to the release of hormones, particularly DHEA (a hormone critical to anti-aging and longevity), can often lead to depletion of vital nutrients in the body, such as vitamin C, and the B-complex vitamins.

During stress, the body overuses its DHEA supply, and thus impairing the normal functioning of its hormonal glands. According to scientific research, an individual's DHEA levels decrease with age. Therefore, stress only adds insult to injury in the aging process.

Another interesting study showed that men who regularly meditate (an anti-stress mental strategy) have significantly more DHEA than those who do not, and the difference is even much more significant in women (maybe women do have more stress than men do).

Stress can accelerate the aging process. According to **Robert Sapolsky**, author of *Zebras Don't Get Ulcers*, people in general lose their capability to cope with stress as they continue to age, due to their tendency to have elevated blood pressure, adversely affecting their hormone secretions.

The Signs and Symptoms of Stress

Are you stressed?

Some typical signs and symptoms of a distressed body and mind may include: aggression and anger; breathing difficulties and problems; indigestion and eating disorders; excess sweating; chronic fatigue; frequent headache; memory loss; muscle tension; poor concentration and indecision, among others.

Remember, stress is one of the key factors contributing to aging. Anxiety and depression—often the byproducts of stress—are often the precursors to autoimmune diseases, such as diabetes and rheumatoid arthritis, among others. By accelerating breathing, elevating blood pressure, and constricting blood flow, stress may also be the culprit of cancers and heart diseases.

The Origin of Stress

Stress originates from the thinking mind. Stress is no more than your perception of your attitude or personal reaction to certain events and experiences in your life. In other words, what is stress to you may not be stress to another person.

William Shakespeare once said: "There is nothing either good or bad, but thinking makes it so." **John Milton**, the famous English poet, also had this to say: "The mind is its own place, and in itself can make Heaven of Hell, a Hell of Heaven." Both spoke volumes of the perceptions of stress.

Therefore, subconscious energies of the mind play a pivotal role in stress management.

The Causes of Stress

Emotional Factors

Anger, bitterness, disappointment, and envy are some of the common human emotions that often lead to anxiety, distress, and even depression.

Environmental and Eventful Factors

A dangerous environment, such as walking alone in the dark or in an unsafe neighborhood, can be stressful.

A work environment with racial discrimination or sexual harassment can be stressful too. According to the American Institute of Stress, up to one million employees' daily absence is mostly stress related. In addition, work environment may create stress due to feeling unproductive, inability to concentrate on work, unrealistic and unreasonable demands from employers or co-workers.

Stressful life events may also lead to elevated stress levels. Special life events—whether they are positive or negative—can be stressful, such as getting married or planning a wedding, graduation, starting a new job, buying a home, or even going on a vacation.

Financial Factors

Finance is one of the main stress factors in contemporary life and living due to rampant unemployment, not having enough money to make both ends meet, debt from credit cards or reckless over-spending, bankruptcy, and home foreclosure.

Health Factors

According to the American Academy of Family Physicians, two-thirds of all family doctor visits are stress related.

Health problems can be triggered by alcohol, sugar, and tobacco addiction. Chronic health problems, such as autoimmune diseases, cancers and heart-related health issues, are particularly stressful after diagnoses and during treatments.

Relationship Factors

Relationships are often a source of emotional and psychological problems, such as breakup in a love relationship, separation and divorce, dealing with teenager problems, and coping with aging parents.

The Anatomy of Stress

Stress may come in different forms: experience of stress can be past, current, and future.

Past stress—also known as "residual stress"—is stress from the past that you have not overcome completely despite the passage of time.

Current stress is a "current state of arousal" caused by an existing situation that requires your immediate attention but that you do not enjoy addressing it.

Future stress is "anticipatory stress or worry" about what might happen in the future. Residual stress can also lead to future stress, passed on from unpleasant past experiences.

Perceptions of stress are generally based on the following: the more you care and value about something, the more stress you have; the more choices and options available to you, the less stress you have; the more conscientious you are, the greater is your stress; the more enjoyment you have, the less stress you feel; and the more responsibility you have, the greater is your stress.

To sum up, stress is all in *your* thinking mind.

TWO

THE CONVENTIONAL WISDOM

Stress has become a serious health issue. Nearly everyone is suffering from some kind of stress every day, whether it is the short-term stress that triggers the human body to reach heightened awareness and preparation for action (what is known as the "fight-or-flight" response), or the devastating long-term chronic stress.

The conventional wisdom has many different ways to help you coping with stress.

Different Medical Systems for Stress Relief

The Conventional Western Medicine

The conventional Western medicine has been using advanced science and technology for diagnosis and treatment of symptoms of diseases or disorders.

All remedies in the conventional Western medicine involve chemicals, some of which are even toxic to human health. In the beginning of the 20th century, Western medical science had dismissed even traditional Western plant remedies as folklore medicine—concoctions only for grandmothers but not for professionally trained doctors. With the emergence of the pharmaceutical industry, Western scientists began to focus almost exclusively on chemical drugs to treat different diseases with different symptoms. A case in point is human cancer. In the early 20th century, cancer was relatively unknown, but the number of cancer cases soon began to explode exponentially. With the growth of the billion-dollar pharmaceutical industry and the need to validate the potency of these chemical drugs, more research studies have to be conducted. Given that Western medicine aims at treating the symptoms rather than at eradicating the root causes of a disease, and that chemical drugs often generate many adverse side effects, more new chemical drugs have to be developed to treat those newly emerging symptoms.

The general approach of the conventional Western medicine is to "cure-all." But, unfortunately, all pharmaceutical drugs, irrespective of their potency in suppressing the symptoms of diseases and disorders, are toxic chemicals that ultimately create more stress in the body system.

Consider the pros and cons of the conventional Western medicine in relieving stress symptoms. The wisdom is to think twice before you reach out for your sleep medications or antidepressants.

The Traditional Chinese Medicine

The Traditional Chinese Medicine (TCM) is based on the wisdom of more than 2,000 years of highly sophisticated techniques of observation and diagnosis of diseases and disorders. This medical system was founded on the concept of balance and harmony (the *yin* and the *yang*) with its focus on diets, herbs, energy healing (acupuncture), and body massage, among others.

The fundamental concept underlying the Chinese medicine is the TAO wisdom, which essentially means that "all things develop naturally" or "one power underlying all." That is to say, all things are what they are, and they come into being as well as decay for what they really are.

The balance and harmony of the *yin* and *yang* is also reflected in the Five Elements (wood, fire, earth, metal, and water) representing the five processes that are not only fundamental to the natural cycles of nature but also corresponding to the different organs of the human body. To illustrate, *wood* feeds on *fire* to produce ashes (*earth*); without which there is no *metal*; the metal inside earth is heated, liquefied by fire to produce *water* through condensation; without water, there is no wood, and hence no fire, no earth, no metal, and no water. Each of the Five Elements is equally important, and each is responsible for the five processes of action and interaction in the cycle of nature, balancing and complementing one another for co-existence and harmony, which is the essence of overall health and wellness, including freedom from stress.

In addition, in the human body, *wood* relates to the

liver (*yin*) and the gall bladder (*yang*); *fire* relates to the heart (*yin*) and the small intestines (*yang*); *earth* relates to the spleen (*yin*) and the stomach (*yang*); *metal* relates to the lungs (*yin*) and the large intestines (*yang*); and *water* relates to the kidneys (*yin*) and the urinary bladder (*yang*). They control and regulate each other for their maintenance, sustenance, and survival.

Furthermore, the Chinese medicine focuses on plants as remedies. Plants are essential to life. In fact, nearly all human food comes from plants or animals that eat plants. Accordingly, in the Chinese medicine, the number of plants used as medicines is greater than the number of plants for food. In the Chinese medicine, there is not much distinction between a food and a medicine. Even thousands of years before Christ, the Chinese believed that every single plant on earth has its specific function in the well-being of an individual.

Unlike the conventional Western medicine, the ultimate objective of the Chinese medicine is to "heal-all."

Consider that stress is about balance and harmony within and without. The wisdom is to live a life of balance and harmony for stress relief.

The Ayurvedic Medicine

The Ayurvedic medicine is based on 5,000 years of the expertise and knowledge of sages in India with respect to health and healing. It is the first medical system in the world. Originally, there were two schools of Ayurveda: the school of physicians and the school of surgeons. Through centuries of transformation, they have now evolved into a scientifically veritable and classifiable medical system widely used in India.

The word "Ayurveda" means "science of life." Therefore, its main focus is on self-discovery with deep meditation to understand the potency of healing through foods, herbs, aromas, gems, colors, massages, and yoga, among others

The wisdom of Ayurveda became the foundation of Buddhism, Taoism, Tibetan and other cultural medicines in the Far East. The essence of the Ayurvedic medicine is self-growth and self-enlightenment to provide many answers to the questions about health and wellness that are all within the self of an individual. After all, nobody knows the self better than oneself. The base for healing is rooted in everyday diet and lifestyle, which play a pivotal role in the health and wellness of the body, the mind, and the soul.

The holistic approach of the Ayurvedic medicine involves three criteria. The first is that one does not just treat a disease but one uses the disease for self-understanding; that is, *why* and *how* one gets the disease in the first place. The second is that one must not follow a general program; instead, one should have a program uniquely catered to the needs of oneself, because what is applicable to one may not be applicable to another. The third is that one should not impose any discipline on oneself to follow the program: the explanation is that any imposition may stimulate one's inherent resistant nature; discovery of one's own sensitivity is more important than rigidity.

The Ayurvedic medicine has a holistic approach to stress relief. The wisdom is to use meditation and yoga for clarity of the mind and fitness of the body for stress relief.

The Alternative and the Complementary Medicine

The alternative medicine is the use of any practice to achieve the healing effects of medicine. It may consist of a wide range of practices, products, procedures, and therapies that have not been scientifically proven to be efficacious. They may include homeopathy (the use of minute doses of a substance to stimulate the body's own self-healing mechanism), as well as naturopathy (acupuncture, massage therapy, and herbal remedies).

The Complementary and Alternative Medicine (CAM) is the use of both the alternative medicine and the conventional Western medicine so that they may help each other to attain the desired healing. Nearly 40 percent of adults report using the Complementary and Alternative Medicine.

The bottom line: the wisdom is to have an empty mind, open to any other options for stress relief.

Stress-Relief Strategies

There are many different strategies for stress relief.

Healthy Lifestyle Strategy

A healthy lifestyle goes a long way to reducing stress. A healthy lifestyle involves giving up alcohol and tobacco. Addiction to these substances is a source of stress for the body, the mind, and the soul.

Alcohol

Alcohol is a depressant. Heavy drinking, in particular, interferes with the neurotransmitters in your brain, and thus damaging your mental health over the long haul.

Kick the habit of instinctively reaching out for a bottle of beer or a glass of wine after a stressful day in the office. Yes, alcohol may help you deal with stress in the short term; in the long term, however, it may contribute to your feeling of depression and anxiety, and thus making your stress even harder to deal with. Worst of all, it may create your addiction that is the ultimate source of stress.

Nicotine

Contrary to the popular belief that nicotine can calm you down, **Jon Kassel**, a psychologist at the University of Illinois at Chicago, stated that "If you're nervous and you're smoking in your home alone, with nothing to distract you, your attention almost becomes more focused on the unpleasant things." Therefore, nicotine may actually *increase* your anxiety.

This is *how*.

Nicotine creates an immediate sense of relaxation so you smoke in the erroneous belief that it may help you reduce your stress and anxiety. Unfortunately, this feeling of relaxation is only temporary, and soon gives way to your withdrawal symptoms and your increased cravings. Smoking reduces nicotine withdrawal symptoms, which are similar to the symptoms of anxiety; therefore, it does not reduce anxiety or deal with the underlying causes.

In addition, nicotine makes you become more vulnerable to depression. Nicotine stimulates the release of the chemical dopamine in your brain, and thereby instrumental in triggering positive feelings. Using cigarettes as a way of temporarily increasing your dopamine supply is unwise because smoking also encourages your brain to switch off its own mechanism for making dopamine. As a result, over the long haul, your brain's supply of dopamine decreases, which in turn prompts you to smoke more.

Healthy eating and drinking

A healthy lifestyle also includes a healthy diet of eating and drinking.

Healthy eating and drinking is the foundation of good health and disease prevention. A healthy diet means eating naturally, which is avoiding as much as possible processed foods and drinks (that is, anything that comes in a box or carton; any energized or fortified drink is unnatural). Always read food labels to see if they contain ingredients that are chemicals or unintelligible to you.

Eat an anti-inflammatory diet. While inflammation is your body's natural mechanism to heal and fight against infection and an overactive immune system, chronic inflammation is now thought to be the underlying cause of multiple health conditions, including cancer, diabetes, heart disease, and obesity. An anti-inflammatory diet contains whole grains, lean protein sources, fresh fruits and vegetables, and nuts. On the other hand, foods high in sugar or saturated fats and trans-fats, deep fried foods, and highly processed foods only induce inflammation, which causes stress to the body and the mind.

Always drink at least eight glasses of water a day. Drinking alcohol and taking pharmaceutical drugs dehydrate the body, and causing undue stress.

Natural Sleep Strategy

Sleep is a natural human instinct. Natural sleep is an essential component of stress-free living.

Research studies have shown that all living things sleep. A Swiss research study indicated that gold fish, having been deprived of sleep for an extended period of time, would stay still for a protracted period of time to make up for its sleep deprivation; and that also applied to cockroaches. In other words, sleep deprivation would only lead to an increased need for sleep later, and all animals need sleep and instinctively know how to sleep. Man is no exception: natural sleep is the essence of his being, without which there is stress.

Unfortunately, sleep insomnia is one of the common sleep disorders. Many people not only have difficulty in getting natural sleep but also have to rely on sleep aids to help them sleep. Indeed, sleep insomnia is a growing health problem in modern society because people are living in a pressure-cooker environment.

Good sleep environment

Good sleep environment not only promotes natural sleep without the use of medication but also makes you sleep better.

Temperature affects your sleep, because your body temperature plays a pivotal part in your sleep process. Your body temperature changes according to your biological clock, which makes you want to sleep. Your body temperature rises in the early evening, and gradually cools down throughout the night until around 4 o'clock in the morning. Accordingly, the temperature of the bedroom and that of your bed must be optimum to induce natural sleep: that is, a temperature in the range of 62°F (16° C) and 71° F (24° C); anything above or below that temperature range may cause restlessness that prevents good natural sleep.

Adjust the humidity of your sleep environment. A too-dry sleep environment may affect your bronchial passages, causing constant coughing, which interrupts deep sleep. To prevent dryness, place a bowl of water to humidify the bedroom environment, especially in winter with the heat on. On the other hand, a too-humid bedroom causes dampness, which may raise your stress hormone levels. To avoid dampness, you may want to have your bed linen made from natural fabrics to help you absorb any perspiration as well as to allow your skin to breathe more freely.

Eating behavior

Eating behavior also contributes to insomnia. Eating increases your metabolic rate as well as your body temperature, which are critical factors in natural sleep. Body temperature dropping is conducive to good sleep. That explains why you should not eat at least three hours before going to bed.

A high body temperature prevents you from falling asleep, not to mention the bloated feeling that may bother you if you eat too much before bedtime. You may also have experienced sluggishness after a heavy lunch meal, but that does not mean you can actually go to sleep faster or sleep better. The explanation is that a heavy meal causes your brain to divert energy from your muscles to work with your digestive system. This may disrupt your brain activities, and thus preventing you from sleeping well.

Generally, it is better to eat smaller meals than to eat one heavy meal with one or two light meals in between. Eating too much at one meal stresses not just your digestive system but also your brain.

Your eating behavior also includes the types of food you consume during the day. Cheese, for example, is said to give nightmares because it contains tyramine, an ingredient in cheese that can elevate blood pressure. MSG (monosodium glutamate), a taste enhancer in most restaurant cuisines, may cause digestive upsets, heartburn, and headaches, which may often interrupt natural sleep. Yellow tartrazine, often added to fizzy drinks, candies, and cookies, may increase hyper-activity that may prevent you from falling asleep fast. In short, foods that damage your health may also impair your sleep health.

Drinking behavior

Many seniors erroneously believe that if they drink too much, they need to frequent the bathroom more often, and thus may affect their sleep patterns. However, dehydration may adversely affect the brain, and hence the ability to sleep well at night. To improve sleep health, drink at least two liters (8 cups) of water a day, and drink it early in the morning so as to avoid bathroom trips at night.

Addiction behavior

To sleep well, avoid smoking or drinking an alcoholic "nightcap."

Nicotine may relax your body and mind, and make you fall asleep faster. However, once the nicotine is metabolized, it will wake you up in the middle of the night. Research studies at the University of Pennsylvania indicated that smokers took twice as long to fall asleep as non-smokers. Quite smoking to benefit both physical and sleep health.

Drinking alcohol may be habit forming. If you have emotional problems, then you must resolve them, instead of using alcohol to obliterate them. If you really need a drink before bedtime, substitute your alcoholic drink with a hot milky drink or herbal drink.

Physical activities

Physical activities, which expand the natural range of movements, may help you sleep well. If your body remains too long in any one position, tension builds up in your muscles, and physical stress causes restlessness that may prevent you from sleeping well. Do pre-sleep stretch exercise to relax muscles and to relieve anxiety to make you sleep faster and better.

But avoid any vigorous physical exercise prior to sleep.

Meditation

Meditation is thinking about one thing at a time. Simple as it is, it requires practice and discipline. According to **St. Theresa of Avila**, the mind is like an unbridled horse wandering where it will, and your role is to train the horse and gently and lovingly bring it back to the right course. Meditation is an effective way to calm your body and mind to prepare you for natural sleep. Meditation releases any blocked energy due to your inadvertent attachment to any thought; by de-cluttering your mind, meditation helps you let go of any restless thoughts that may prevent you from sleeping well. (Also go to **Meditation and Mindfulness Strategy** below.)

To sum up, if you are suffering from insomnia, there must be a health issue that needs to be addressed. Use your mind power through subliminal messages (go to **Affirmations and Visualization Strategy** below) to ease your insomnia by targeting negative thoughts, distorted patterns of thinking, and blockages deep within your subconscious mind. These subliminal messages may help you sleep by relaxing your body, calming your mind, and slowing down your thoughts, so as to ease you off to sleep. In addition, these subliminal messages may also permanently rewire your subconscious mind to eliminate your insomnia forever.

Problem Solving Strategy

If you have problems, solve them. Solving problems requires intention and decision, perseverance and persistence, commitment and dedication. It is not easy, but doable. Procrastination, which is the major obstacle to problem solving strategy, is also the source of stress.

The major life problems are related to career, money, relationship, adversity, and time (more on these in **Part Four**).

Career problems

Your career may span over decades, involving many ups and downs, such as promotion and unemployment, changes of career and pursuits of higher qualifications, among others. Their related problems need to be resolved to relieve the related stress.

Money problems

Money plays a major role in life. You need money

for almost everything in life. Given the importance of money, you need to know the basics of money—what money is all about.

In the past, people could enjoy the blessings of life without spending any *real* money. Nowadays, to many people, enjoyment of life requires money—and lots of it!

According to **Buddha**, craving or desire for material things is the fountainhead of all human miseries. **Jesus** also has this to say about money: "It is easier for a camel to pass through the eye of a needle than for a rich man to go to heaven." (**Luke** 18:25)

So, what is the *value* of money? According to author **Jonathan Swift**, a wise man should have money in his head, but not in his heart.

More importantly, what does money mean to *you*?

Your perceptions of the *value* of money determine two of the most important things in your life: how you are going to *live* your life; how you are going to *spend* your money.

The value of money is based on your *core values* in life. One of the core values in life is *integrity*. Life, at any phase, is all about *living*—it comes with some hard work and simple integrity. Integrity is an important personal value, which has little to do with money. Integrity is an important value that the Creator has bestowed on each and every one of us, and its availability is the choice of an individual. Essentially, integrity is the *value of what life has to offer*, not the value of things that can be purchased with money. Your core values affect your *attitudes* toward money, including your financial priorities, financial decisions, and money management. So, what is the value of money to *you*?

Once you know the *real* value of money to you, you will know what to do with your money, and you will find the money you need.

Spending money is also an extremely important issue in life: throughout history, countries have become bankrupt, empires have collapsed, and families have broken up because of spending much too much money. So, spending money can affect positively or negatively your life, and can be a major stress factor.

Spending money has little to do with whether you have or you do not have much money. Spending money has to do with your *attitude* toward money. It has everything to do with the *practical* as well as the *spiritual* aspects of money and finance.

The *practical* aspect of spending money is that it may lead to *debt*—which is the source of financial stress.

Why do people go into debt?

People go into debt for various reasons: *deficit*

spending, a result of buying things they do not need with the money they do not have; *unforeseeable circumstances*, due to exorbitant medical bills or unemployment; *personal choice*, a consequence of reckless spending or buying on credit, bad investments, wrong financial decisions; *ignorance*, such as not knowing the meaning of APR or the implications of "minimum payments" on credit cards, lack of knowledge of finance and money management; *greed*, leading to taking financial risks, or trying to get something for nothing. The list could go and on.

Don't ever fall into the trap of "buy-now-and-pay-later"! Don't run up your credit card debt. Consumer debt is the No.1 financial stress factor in life. Don't let debt devastate your life. Don't use a credit card if you don't have control over spending; instead, use a debit card or a pre-paid credit card for the convenience of not carrying cash. Be careful when you use credit-card counseling services to get you out of debt, especially those so-called "non-profit" organizations. Just beware!

The *spiritual* aspects of spending money include being grateful and generous, as well as being a good steward.

Be grateful. God may have given you *much less* than others—or so you think! Just remember that everything is *relative*. Maybe less is *more*: God has given you *less* so that you will have the incentive to make *more*.

You may have worked hard, but with little to show for it. "You plant much but harvest little. You have scarcely enough to eat or drink and not enough to keep you warm. Your income disappears, as though you were putting it into pockets filled with holes." (**Haggai** 1:6) Be grateful, instead of whining and complaining; put your time and effort on making money to live a debt-free life. More importantly, be generous with your money.

According to the Biblical principle of money, God owns it all! You are but a steward of God's money. Responsibilities of good stewardship may include diligence, productivity, good time management, and self-discipline in matters of money. The money is not yours anyway. That is why you cannot take it with you when you are gone for good.

Relationship problems

Living has to do with people, involving agreement and disagreement—often a source of conflict and stress.

Harmonious human relationships require knowledge of the self and others; that is, a deep understanding of who you are as well as of others around you through positive mentality with your love and compassion.

To act with positive mentality, you need to evaluate your own emotions to see how positive or negative they may be. This will help you act with the right mentality.

Emotional intelligence is the use of mental skill to understand, perceive, and explain human emotions and feelings in order to promote better thinking and to enhance better and greater cognitive activities. Most importantly, emotional intelligence helps you manage your own emotions in a positive way, as well as enables you to lead a happier life through improved relationships with others around you.

Emotional intelligence plays a pivotal role in human life. All human organs, tissues, and cells have their respective energetic frequencies, which are quite different from those of negative emotions and thoughts. Therefore, it is critical that you fully and appropriately experience and process your negative emotional energies, lest they get trapped inside your body and mind, causing long-term health hazards and relationship problems. Therefore, it is critical that you are able to identify, utilize, understand, and manage your emotions as well as those in others around you for stress relief, effective communication, and diffusion of conflicts. In short, emotional intelligence plays a pivotal role in your relationships with others.

Enhance your emotional intelligence, which is all about your awareness, control, and management of emotions. Very often you just experience your own emotions and react to them without any awareness, and this is where the problem lies. Therefore, to enhance your emotional intelligence, you must begin with your awareness, which is your mental concentration. Awareness is the recognition of your own emotions and how they may affect your behavior and thinking, positively or negatively, as well as the knowledge of your own strength and weakness in how you react to those emotions.

With awareness, you begin to acquire the capability to control and restrain your own compulsive feelings and behaviors, such as your commitment to delaying reactions and your willingness to adapting to changing the circumstances in your life.

With awareness, you may also have a better understanding of the emotions of others around you. In their shoes, you may have more empathic feelings of why and how they behave or react in certain ways. Empathy is your connection with other human beings, which is critical to maintaining good human relationships.

Dalai Lama, the Tibetan spiritual leader, demonstrates how he instantly connects to people of different cultures, religions, and perspectives. Accordingly, on the very first meeting with any individual, he trains himself to feel that the individual is simply "a fellow human being with the same desire to be happy and to avoid suffering as myself." With that mindset, he becomes "connected" to everybody, without any exception.

C.S. Lewis, author and intellectualist, shows how

you can "discipline" your negative emotions. When you know that you are not going to behave friendly toward another person, *consciously* put on a more friendly manner, such as a big smile, and behave as if you were a much nicer person than you actually are. In a few minutes, you may actually *feel* friendlier toward that person.

In short, cherishing the attributes of emotional intelligence will enhance your own emotional intelligence to become a better person and to develop better relationships with others.

Adversity problems

In the course of human life, loss and bereavement are as inevitable as death. Loss is a life changer, changing the course and direction of the life journey one is embarking on, without which life becomes static, and a static life is meaningless and not worth living. Loss can be physical, material, and even spiritual, such as loss of hope and purpose.

Accepting, embracing, and letting go hold the key to recovery and rejuvenation from any adversity in life. In addition, one may learn a valuable life lesson from any adversity encountered in life. Your perspective of any adversity is often the solution to that adversity problem.

Right Breathing Strategy

Breathing gives life. Without food and water, you

may still survive for a while, but without your breath, you die within minutes.

Breathing has to do with the lungs, which serve two main functions: to get life-giving oxygen from the air into the body, and to remove toxic carbon dioxide from the body. So, do not compromise your lung functions with nicotine.

Breathing patterns are critical to health. That is, *how* you breathe may positively or negatively affect your body organs and hormones. For example, taking short, shallow breaths, you are in fact telling your brain that a threat exists, which then stimulates a stress response, and thus creating destructive thinking patterns in your brain. Conversely, taking long, deep breaths you are sending positive signals to your brain for positive thinking patterns. When you own your breath, you have calm and peace. Breathing is just a simple strategy for instant stress relief.

Diaphragm breathing

Learn how to breathe right: diaphragm breathing.

Diaphragm breathing is the *complete* breath. Consciously change your breathing patterns. Use your diaphragm to breathe (the diaphragm muscle separating your chest from your abdomen). Place one hand on your breastbone, feeling that it is raised, and put the other hand above your waist, feeling the diaphragm muscle moving up and down.

Deep breathing with your diaphragm gives you complete breath. This is how you do diaphragm breathing:

- Sit comfortably.
- Begin your slow exhalation through your nose.
- Contract your abdomen to empty your lungs.
- Begin your slow inhalation and simultaneously make your belly bulge out.
- Continuing your slow inhalation, now, slightly contract your abdomen and simultaneously lift your chest and hold.
- Continue your slow inhalation, and slowly raise your shoulders. This allows the air to enter fully into your lungs to attain the complete breath.
- Retain your breath and slightly raise your shoulders for a count of 5.
- Very slowly exhale the air. Your upper chest deflates first, and then your abdomen relaxes in.
- Repeat the process.

Learn to slowly prolong your breath, especially your exhalation. Relax your chest and diaphragm muscle, so that you can extend your exhalation, making your breathing out longer and complete. To prolong your exhalation, count "one-and-two-and-three" as you breathe in and breathe out. Make sure that they become balanced. Once you have mastered that, then try to make your breathing out a little longer than your breathing in.

Practice diaphragm breathing until it becomes second nature to you. Diaphragm breathing is relaxing and stress relieving.

Alternate-nostril breathing

Alternate-nostril breathing is a basic Yoga breathing exercise to balance the right side and the left side of your brain. This exercise is especially ideal for enhancing your body balance, as well as internal harmony and stress relief.

The left side of your brain governs the right side of your body, including your speech and logical thinking, while the right side of your brain governs the left side of your body, including your creativity and intuition. Achieving balance and harmony between the two sides of your brain is critical to mind healing for deep relaxation and stress relief. You can balance your mental energy from the right and the left side of the brain while practicing your alternate-nostril breathing during meditation or a mind-relaxation session. Practice alternate-nostril breathing everyday for stress relief.

This is how to practice alternate-nostril breathing:

- Place your thumb and ring finger lightly on your right and your left nostrils, respectively, with your index and middle fingers resting lightly on your forehead just between your eyebrows.

- Exhale deeply through BOTH nostrils.
- Press your thumb against the RIGHT nostril to CLOSE it.
- Breathe in through your LEFT nostril. Count 8.
- CLOSE your LEFT nostril by pressing down your ring finger. Now, BOTH nostrils are closed. Retain the air, and count 4.
- OPEN your RIGHT nostril, and breathe out. Count 8.
- With the LEFT nostril still CLOSED, breathe in through the RIGHT nostril. Count 8.
- CLOSE the RIGHT nostril. Now, BOTH nostrils are closed. Retain the air, and count 4.
- OPEN the LEFT nostril, and breathe out with the RIGHT nostril still closed. Count 8.
- With the RIGHT nostril closed, you have breathed out through the LEFT nostril; you have now completed one round of the breathing exercise.
- Begin the second round by breathing in through the LEFT nostril, and repeat the above.

Here is a short summary of alternative-nostril breathing:

- Breathe out through BOTH nostrils. .
- Breathe in through the LEFT nostril (count 8).
- Close BOTH nostrils, and retain the air (count 4).
- Breathe out through the RIGHT nostril (count

8).

- Breathe in through the RIGHT nostril (count 8).
- Close BOTH nostrils, and retain the air (count 4).
- Breathe out through the LEFT nostril (count 8).
- Breathe in through the LEFT and repeat the whole process.

Practice your alternate-nostril breathing to create acute awareness and concentration, as well as to enhance your internal body balance to *de*-stress yourself.

Affirmations and Visualization Strategy

Life is an unfathomable mystery. If everything in your life is dead certain, then there is no mystery any more, and most probably your life is one of mediocrity. You certainly would like your life to be more exciting, and making more new waves. Your pains and sufferings, trials, and tribulations—they can actually be your spring-boards to overwhelming happiness, if you would let your mind function in the right way by controlling and manipulating your thoughts.

Affirmations

Affirmations are positive subliminal messages sent directly to your subconscious mind, which controls your conscious mind. Use subliminal messages to *consciously control* what you may be doing all day long and everyday—thinking *uncreatively* and *unintelligently*.

According to **Albert Einstein**, any man who reads too much and uses his own brain too little falls into the lazy habits of thinking. You may *think* you are thinking, but in fact you are not because you have developed the lazy habits of thinking. As a matter of fact, the vast majority of people in this world do not even do their own thinking, much less creating their own subliminal messages in their minds. They do not know what they are thinking, and they do not know what they are feeling, because they do not know *how* to visualize their future.

Affirmations are powerful mental tools to enhance your mind. Empower your mind with subliminal messages, which work as a mild form of self-hypnosis—slowly and gradually sending positive suggestions into your subconscious mind to subtly change any incorrect self-beliefs, wrong ways of thinking, and even undesirable patterns of behavior.

Affirmations enable you not only to bypass your "logical" conscious mind but also to overcome any resistance that may hold you back, thereby enabling you to access your subconscious mind with positive messages to enhance your mind power. Subliminal messages are powerful tools to empower your mind to live a much better life free from stress.

Once you have mastered the subliminal messages, you can master your mind by controlling its thoughts. Remember, you are your thoughts, and your life is a byproduct of all your thoughts. As **Napoleon Hill**, the famous writer, said: "What the mind of man can conceive and believe, it can achieve." Yes, you can achieve what your mind has set out to accomplish—a stress-free life.

How to use affirmations

You must use positive words about yourself and not someone else. Always use "I" in your affirmations because they are all about you and not someone else, for example, "I am happy!" You must use the present tense as if you are speaking to your mind right now, for example, "I am now relaxed!"

You must prompt your subconscious mind to remember the things you want, not the things you don't. For example, do not say: "I am now going to give up alcohol!" because your subconscious mind registers "alcohol" which is what you would want to give up; instead, say: "I am now going to be calm and sober!"

You must always be positive, and not the reverse of a negative, for example, "I am not stressed." Instead, say: "I am calm, relaxed, and peaceful."

You must repeat your subliminal messages only when you are mentally relaxed, and you must repeat them consistently and diligently to achieve the desired effect.

Visualization

Visualization is a powerful mental tool to help you achieve your goal of freedom from stress. Visualize your future self in your mind's eye. A picture is worth a thousand words. If you can imagine it, you can achieve it. According to **Albert Einstein**, your imagination is much more important than your knowledge.

Harness the power of visualization to make it more "real" to you, and this gives you the incentive to pursue your freedom from stress. Visualization is manifestation of your desires by vibrating their mental energy frequencies in a positive way.

How to visualize

You must be very relaxed; your mind must be in a deep level of relaxation. You must "strongly feel" that you have already got what you want, not just "thinking" about getting what you want. Remember, "wanting" is the opposite of "having." The former generates negative energy frequencies, while the latter creates positive ones. Positive feelings are a key component of visualization.

You must visualize with your specific details to authenticate the reality of your visualization. For example, when visualizing how relaxed you are, you see in your mind's eye how you are lying on the beach, listening to the soft sound of waves lapping against the sandy shore, while sipping your favorite drink and looking up at the cloudless blue sky.

You must be in full control. A positive image stems from an internal focus of control, which means you always act instead of reacting, and you are always the master of a situation, instead of the victim, worrying about its possible negative outcome.

You must be consistent in your visualization. Your mind is a muscle; you must exercise it constantly and consistently to create the desirable strength to accomplish its mission.

You must be patient with your visualization. You must think long term; that is, you must patiently wait for the manifestation of your goals visualized.

Meditation and Mindfulness Strategy

Meditation is a mind-control exercise aimed at improving the quality of thinking. There is nothing mystical or religious about meditation; it is only a myth that it is both. Meditation is simply a state of mind—more specifically, a *mindful* state of the mind, in which there is deep body-mind relaxation with the inexplicable experiences of peace and tranquility. A meditative mind is just intense presence of the mind, or mindfulness of the present moment to the exclusion of everything else.

Why meditate?

Given that meditation is a non-doing state of your

mind in which you consciously cherish and cultivate a relationship with your inner world, meditation is instrumental in fixing many of your daily life problems. Having said that, it must be pointed out that using medication solely to fix your life problems is not going to work. Instead, use meditation to befriend yourself, to know more about who you are, and to convey love and compassion to others, thereby instrumental in fixing some of your life problems. Meditation is only a means to an end, but not an end in itself. Therefore, it is important not to meditate with *any* expectation: it defeats the purpose of meditation, which is internalization of the self with no expectation.

The mind slows down only during sleep, during which it never completely rests. One of the objectives of meditation is to slow down the thinking mind, while increasing its total awareness (this is where it differs from sleep in which the mind slows down and its awareness is concurrently reduced to a minimum) through enhanced concentration, which is mental awareness of the present moment. In short, mindfulness is full awareness of what is happening at the present moment.

Remember, anything you focus on during meditation will bring you into the present moment, giving you the very experience of "presence" of your mind.

According to recent scientific studies, after several months of intense meditation training, participants demonstrated two significant changes in their minds: increase in brain chemicals responsible for increased happiness; enhancement of mental perceptions to uncover more details about their past.

Another benefit of meditation is that you do not need to know how the brain works in order to meditate or develop mindfulness. The ultimate purpose of meditation is to let your mind stay in a state of mindfulness in which you are more relaxed with clarity of mind and thinking to become a more loving human being.

How to meditate

Find a quiet place where you can remain undisturbed for 10 to 30 minutes. To set the environment for meditation, you may want to have some scent from flowers or incense, or even some soothing music (meditation MP3) to enhance your senses. Of course, you can meditate without any of them; it is just an option, not a requirement.

Find time to practice meditation. Regularity holds the key to success in meditation. Do not meditate only when you feel like it. Find some quiet time for yourself every day. The ideal time to meditate is before retiring to bed; in that way, your mind can review what has happened during the day—what you have said and done—and let go of everything. After all, meditation is about letting go of the past and future thoughts.

Correct posture is important. Firstly, your body must be as erect as possible: this induces correct breathing, which can bring all your internal energies into a state of harmony. Therefore, do not lean back on anything. If you find that your neck is too week and that your spine cannot support your body, then rest your back on a hard surface initially; but the ultimate goal is to sit erect without your back touching anything.

You can sit cross-legged on the floor. Alternatively, you can sit comfortably on a chair (not a sofa), with your thighs at right angles to your spine, your hands on your thighs, your feet resting firmly on the floor, and your shoulders relaxed. In short, just sit "tall" and erect.

Begin meditation with your breathing. Your breathing is an indicator of your stress level: if you are unduly stressed, your breathing becomes thick and gasping. Breathing right is your conscious control of stress. Whenever you feel stressed, consciously change your breathing pace to undo the stress.

Gently close your eyes, or you can fix your eyes on an object close by.

As you begin your meditation, you will find that your first thought does not come to your mind right away. When it finally comes, do not dismiss it. Instead, consciously focus on your breathing. That thought will then slowly disappear. After a while, another thought or the same thought may come up to your mind. Again, do not consciously dismiss it; refocus on your breathing. With more practice, you will find that within a 10-minute time frame, fewer and fewer thoughts will crop up in your mind because your mind has stayed in the present moment for a longer period. The fewer thoughts you have, the more relaxed you become. Then, one day, you may suddenly find that you have stepped into a different world with total tranquility and clarity of mind—even though it may last but a very brief moment. That sensation is nondescript. Once you have attained that inexplicable and transformative state of mind, you will want to continue practicing meditation every day. But do not expect that transcendental state will come any time soon; the more you expect it, the longer it will take you to attain that state of mind. Just consistently and patiently practice meditation every day.

Mindfulness

Mindfulness is acute mental awareness, which is deep concentration of the body and the mind for their interconnection: the body is created to support the mind. To sharpen your mind power, you must enhance the awareness of your body *first*. If you feel that your body, mind, and soul are not connected, most probably there is lack of body awareness by the mind in the first place. Therefore, mental awareness begins with awareness of the body first.

Most of us do not pay much attention to the body—except when we experience physical pain—let alone paying attention to the mind. But mental attention is important to the wisdom in stress-free living. The mind and the body are interconnected. Your mental attention is essentially your body consciousness or your attention to the physical conditions and the needs of your body in relation to how your mind thinks. Understanding this intricate relationship may help you relax both your body and mind.

Are you always paying conscious attention to your body at all times? The way you normally eat speaks volumes of the degree or intensity of your body awareness. It is not the food you eat, but *how* you are eating your food that shows your body awareness. While eating, if you are reading your newspaper, watching your TV, working on your computer, or checking your cell phone, you are not paying *any* attention to your body, which at that very moment is supposed to be eating and not doing multitasking.

Train your mind to pay more attention to how your body reacts when you are eating, such as chewing your food thoroughly, slowing down your eating process by tasting each morsel of the food in your mouth. Always give your full presence of your mind to your meal. Again, how often you look at something without seeing it at all because your mind is not paying its full attention to what you are looking at. When your mind is not paying its full attention, your body becomes incapacitated; only when your body becomes fully conscious, then your mental capacity will become enhanced and sharpened. Body awareness is simply paying full attention to what your body is doing at that present moment. In other words, be conscious of what your body is doing when you are eating, walking, or doing anything routine. In any life situation, even while doing your dishes, you can use total body awareness to switch off your thinking mind, and give it a meaningful break for your stress relief.

Exercise Strategy

Exercise in almost any form can relieve stress because it can boost your feel-good endorphins and distract you from daily worries that cause stress.

Nearly any form of exercise, from aerobics to yoga, can act as a stress reliever. Even if you are old and decrepit, or downright out of shape, you can still make a little exercise go a long way toward your stress management.

There is a close connection between exercise and stress relief—and a good reason why exercise should be your stress-relief strategy. Removing your daily tensions through movement and physical activity may, surprisingly, help you focus on a single task with more energy and greater optimism, resulting in making you remain calm with greater clarity of mind in everything that you do. Yes, regular exercise can increase your self-confidence and lower any symptom you may have associated with depression and anxiety. In addition, regular exercise can improve your sleep, which is often disrupted by stress, depression and anxiety.

Walking

Walk to *de*-stress as if everything is a miracle. Yes, walking can *de*-stress you, provided you are mindful of *how* you walk.

Walking is one of the most common exercises because it is simple and easy to do—you just walk. You may walk to your workplace or any destination, or you simply walk as a physical exercise. But walking is more than a physical activity that promotes your physical health; walking can also enhance your mind power to help you cope with your everyday stress—if you have the know-how.

Most of us just walk with our feet, but without fully utilizing the exercise of walking to benefit the mind, because walking is so automatic and mechanical that we no longer pay any attention to our walking. In other words, we don't concentrate when we are walking or doing the exercise of walking. We are so caught up with our destination—such as attending a meeting, or going shopping—that we have no awareness of the process of walking. Many of us have put our feet on automatic pilot, and we are just walking like a robot.

So, how to walk to relieve stress?

When walking, first and foremost, pay attention to your breaths: your breathing in and breathing out, as well as the intensity of your breaths. Next, pay attention to the sensations of your body, such as the feelings of your soles and toes as your shoes touch the ground. Also, pay attention to the shifting of your body weight as you move from your right foot to your left foot. Just be mindful of what is happening to your body as you are walking. The objective of mindfulness walking is to stop your thinking mind for deep relaxation to *de*-stress yourself. It is just like walking meditation

Yoga

Yoga is one of the best exercises for stress relief. Yoga health is holistic health—it involves the body, the mind, and the soul.

The practice of yoga exercise or yoga posture requires setting goals—just as you must set goals for your daily tasks. Yoga practice is manifested in good daily routines, which reinforce diligence, consistency, and even perseverance—attributes in success in anything you do, including stress relief.

Yoga breathing, yoga exercise, and yoga posture all focus on *awareness*. Yoga health trains you to become more mindful of what you are doing in the now, especially as you begin each day. Many people have no clue as to what they are doing during their morning rush. But if you practice yoga health, whether it is yoga breathing, yoga exercise or yoga posture—even for just 10 to 15 minutes—you will achieve a peaceful mindset and a relaxed body through your deep concentration on how you *breathe*, including the rhythm of your breath, or how you *stretch* each part of your body. Yoga health simply trains you to become more aware of every single part of your body, both externally and internally. Yoga health is self-awareness that develops good routines, including a healthy diet and lifestyle.

Indeed, today, many people use yoga as a means of mental training through good daily routines to achieve their goals to lose weight or to manage their stress. Develop that yoga discipline to create your good daily routines in order to achieve your stress management.

Weight training

Studies have shown that weight training in doing leg presses and squats not just improves your leg muscles—it boosts your body's natural production of hormones to increase your muscle mass and strength, as well as your mental alertness free from any stress.

Weight training can be performed with state-of-the-art equipment, or just simply using dumbbells to do routines and exercises to get the same results. The choice is yours.

Herbs and Plants Strategy

For thousands of years, herbs and plants have been used as medicines and therapies for not only healing but also stress relief.

Aromatherapy

Aromatherapy is one of the oldest self-healing arts that uses essentials oils from plants to heal the body, the mind, and the soul for holistic self-healing. The aroma from the essential oils of certain plants through the busting of their tiny glands has therapeutic self-healing effects. The explanation is that these plants, having accumulated the radiant energy from the sun, produce essential oils that have anti-fungal and anti-inflammatory properties. They are effective in stress relief.

Essential oils can be classified according to their rate of evaporation. The high-volatility essential oils (evaporating quickly) have invigorating properties, while the low-volatility essential oils (evaporating more slowly) have calming and sedating properties.

Essential oils do not have any side effects. Quite the contrary, they have salubrious effects on your health and wellness. Their subtle therapeutic effects are conducive to self-healing because they can relax the nervous system, giving clarity of mind for stress control. In addition, they can stimulate the blood circulation to promote better brain and heart health, as well as to calm and sedate perturbed emotions for emotional health.

Aroma goes through the nose to the brain, thereby positively affecting the limbic system of the brain for optimum emotional health and calmness of the mind for stress relief.

To illustrate, the aroma of sweet orange oil is conducive to calming the nerves and enhancing emotional balance that may lead to positive outlook. The smell of lavender oil is also effective in overcoming winter blues.

Herb therapy

Herbs have been around for thousands of years for cure and healing. The medicinal values of many herbs have been validated by many research studies. As a result, the interest in herbal cures has soared for many reasons: herbs are often safer than pharmaceutical drugs, which are toxic chemicals; herbs have fewer side effects because they are gentler than many conventional drugs; herbs are natural because they come from natural plants, and thus providing many options to a pharmaceutical drug.

In the past, back in medieval times, when there was no Saturday's break, life was stressful. In those days, monks who also doubled as doctors put stressed patients on bed of *chamomile* to rest as well as to calm them down. You can also drink *chamomile* tea three times a day to calm your nerves. *Valerian*, *passionflower*, and *skullcap* are some of the most common herbs that you can take in tea, capsule, tincture, or extract for stress relief.

Psychotherapy Strategy

Stress may lead to other mental disorders, such as panic attacks, obsessive thoughts, unrelenting worries, or an incapacitating phobia.

Unlike medication treatments, psycho therapies treat more than just the symptoms of the problem: they can help you uncover the underlying causes of your worries and fears; they teach you how to relax, how to evaluate situations in new perspectives, and how to develop better coping and problem-solving skills and strategies.

There are different therapies for stress relief. Cognitive behavioral therapy (CBT) is the most widely-used therapy for the treatment of stress-related panic disorder, phobias, social anxiety disorder, and generalized anxiety disorder, among many other conditions.

Cognitive behavioral therapy (CBT) addresses negative patterns and distortions in the way we look at the world and ourselves. This therapy involves two main components: the cognitive therapy that examines how negative thoughts contribute to stress; the behavior therapy that examines how behavior and reaction may result in stress.

Essentially, your thoughts rather than external events generate your negative feelings that lead to stress; that is, it is the thinking, and not the circumstances, that causes stress. Therefore, the solution is recognition of those negative feelings manifested in the body, and thus learning coping skills and relaxation techniques to counteract the perceived stress. In addition, it may also involve actual confrontation of stress (what is known as exposure therapy) in real life or in the imagination.

Thoughts of Wisdom

Wisdom is the capability to self-intuit what you already know and then diligently apply it to your everyday life and living. Knowledge is accumulation of facts and information, while wisdom is the connection of these dots to see their logic and relevance in real life situations. For example, a scientist is often knowledgeable in his or her field of specialty, but that scientist may not necessarily be wise in everyday life and living.

In addition, wisdom has much to do with asking questions, which is introspection, a process of self-reflection, without which there is no self-awareness and hence no personal growth and development. A static life is never a life well lived. Therefore, asking questions is self-empowering wisdom—a life-skill tool necessary for the art of living stress free.

Why is that?

It is because the kind of questions you ask determines the kind of life you are going to live. Your questions often trigger a set of mental answers, which may lead to actions or inactions, based on the choices you make from the answers you have obtained. Remember, your life is always the sum of all the choices you have made or going to make in the process.

The Burning Questions

To get the wisdom to cope with stress, ask yourself the following burning questions:

- Do all the above strategies, techniques and tools to cope with your stress work for *you*?
- If they do, then *why* is stress still a universal problem?
- If they work for some, why don't they work for *you*?

The Jigsaw Puzzle

Coping with stress is a very complex and complicated process, just like playing a jigsaw puzzle game: you have to put all the pieces together. All those strategies, techniques, and tools outlined above for stress relief, much like different jigsaw puzzle pieces, have to be juggled before they can all fit in to form the whole piece.

The reason why you may still feel stressed is that

there is one piece missing in your jigsaw puzzle. Without that missing piece, the jigsaw puzzle is forever incomplete and unfinished.

Now, *where* do you find that missing piece of jigsaw puzzle?

That piece of missing jigsaw puzzle is *inside* you. But to find that piece of missing jigsaw puzzle, you need wisdom—not the conventional wisdom, but the unconventional ancient wisdom of the TAO. With the TAO, you may then discover the origin of your stress, or the missing jigsaw puzzle piece. That discovery is your ultimate enlightenment.

THREE

THE TAO

What is the TAO?

The Chinese word "TAO" (道) literally means "path" or "way." The term "the Way" has come to be known as "the path to wisdom." It derives from the ancient classic: *Tao Te Ching* (道 德 經)— in Chinese, "Te" (德) means "virtuosity" and "Ching" (經) means "classic"—which is an ancient Chinese classic written around 6th century B.C. by the sage **Lao Tzu** (meaning "Old Master").

Tao Te Ching has become one of the most translated works in world literature, probably ranking with the Bible as one of the top ten in popularity. This book has altogether 81 very short chapters written in exactly 5,000 words with no punctuation mark. All the punctuation marks in the text were subsequently added by scholars over the centuries.

According to the legend, Lao Tzu was born with gray hair (a sign of wisdom related with old age and experience). He was well known for his profound wisdom. At the city gate, riding backward on an ox, he was detained and "forced" to put down his brilliant ideas in writing before he was allowed to leave China for Tibet. Reluctantly, he put down his profound wisdom in only 5,000 words. That was how *Tao Te Ching* came into existence.

Over the centuries, extracts from his immortal classic have been quoted, explained, interpreted, and translated into multiple languages worldwide because of the controversy and the profound wisdom of its content and language.

Below is my own interpretation and translation of the 81 short chapters of *Tao Te Ching*:

Tao Te Ching

Chapter 1: The Creator

If His ways could be explained or understood,
the Creator would no longer be infinite.
If He had a name or an identity,
the Creator would no longer be eternal.

Being infinite and eternal,
the Creator is the origin of all things.
Once given a name and an identity,
mankind is only the source of all things.

Ever humble, we see the mysteries of all things created.
Ever proud, we see only the manifestations of all things created.

Only the mysteries, and not the manifestations,
show us the Way to true wisdom.

Chapter 2: Dualistic Existence

With the fall of man, good cannot exist without evil.
Man is born with virtues, but grows up with vices.

Likewise, life and death complement each other.
Heaven is eternal life; hell is everlasting death.
Human existence is therefore dualistic:
it can make heaven out of hell, or hell out of heaven.

Faith and lack of faith go along with each other.
The first will be the last, and the last will be the first.

Chapter 3: An Empty Mind for Everything

Focusing on status gives us pride, and not humility.
Hoarding worldly riches deprives us of heavenly assets.

An empty mind, with no craving and no expectation,
helps us let go of everything.
Being in the world and not of the world, we attain heavenly grace.

With heavenly grace, we become pure and selfless.
And everything settles into its own perfect place.

Chapter 4: Heavenly Grace

Heavenly grace is like a well of water,
free to all, just for the asking.
It is inexhaustible: the bounty of eternal life.

It quenches all human thirst:
the thirst for anger, desires, and vengeance.
Thirsty no more, we find peace and heavenly grace.

It is hidden, but forever present.
It is inconceivable and intangible.
It comes from the Creator, the origin of all things.

Chapter 5: No Judgment, No Preference

The Creator has no judgment, and no preference:
He treats everything and everyone alike.
Every manifestation attests to the mysteries of His creation.

So, we, too, embrace everything and everyone with no judgment, and no preference.
His grace, never depleting and forever replenishing, shows us the Way.
Judgment and preference separate us from His grace, causing attachment.
Only with His grace do we find renewal and rebirth along the Way.

Chapter 6: The Identity of the Spirit

The Spirit is as immortal as the Creator.
As the soul of all creations, the Spirit is within the Creator.
As the essence of godliness, the Spirit is like the mother of all.
Its true identity is forever intact and intangible.

It is always present in the hearts of the humble.
It brings perfection because it endures and is eternal.

Chapter 7: The Watcher and Observer

The Creator seems elusive amid the changes of life.
At times, He seems to have forsaken His creations.
In reality, He is simply observing the comings and goings of their follies.

Likewise, we watch the comings and goings
of our likes and dislikes, of our desires and fears.
But we do not identify with them.
With no judgment and no preference,
we see the mysteries of creation.

Chapter 8: Be Like Water

The Spirit is just like water flowing to all things.
Its true nature is to give life indiscriminately to all.
It flows to low places, where people reject and despise.
It flows like a river, nurturing everything and everyone on its way.
Its final stop is the ocean, which is its very origin.

Living by the Spirit, we choose a simple and humble lifestyle.
We meditate to enhance our spirituality.
We love our neighbors as ourselves.
We express compassion to all.
We speak with truth and sincerity.

We live in the present moment.
We take action only when necessary.

Without much ado or over-doing, we trust the guidance of the Spirit.
In this manner, life flows like water, fulfilling itself and also everything naturally.

Chapter 9: Letting Go

Letting go is emptying the mundane,
to be filled with heavenly grace.

Blessed is he who has an empty mind.
He will be filled with knowledge and wisdom from the Creator.
Blessed is he who has no attachment to worldly things.
He will be compensated with heavenly riches.
Blessed is he who has no ego-self.
He will be rewarded with humility to connect with the Creator.
Blessed is he who has no judgment of self and others.
He will find contentment and empathy in everyone.

Letting go of everything is the Way to the Creator.

Chapter 10: The Challenge

Can we embrace both good fortunes and misfortunes in life?
Can we breathe as easily as innocent babies?

Can we see the world created as it is without judgment?
Can we accept both the desirable and the undesirable?
Can we express compassion to all without being boastful?
Can we watch the comings and goings of things without being perturbed?

Saying "yes" to all of the above is spiritual wisdom from the Creator,
who watches the comings and goings in the world He created.

Chapter 11: The Invisible and the Intangible

The spokes and the hub are the visible parts of a wheel.
Clay is the visible material of a pot, which is useful because it contains.
Walls, doors, and windows are visible parts of a house.

We always look for the visible and the tangible without.
But what really matters is the invisible and the intangible within.

Chapter 12: The Mysteries of What Is Within

The more we look, the less we see.
The more we hear, the less we listen.
The more we crave, the crazier we become.

What is materialistic is separate from what is spiritualistic.
Therefore, value what is within, and not what is without.

Chapter 13: Success and Failure

Success and failure are no more than expressions of the human condition.
So, accept both gracefully and willingly, with no judgment, and no preference.
The Creator loves us unconditionally, irrespective of our success or failure.
What is meant by "accept both gracefully and willingly"?
Success is avoiding failure; avoiding failure is seeking success.
Both originate from fear and pride: the sources of human suffering.

Seeing ourselves indiscriminately as everything, including success and failure,
we see not only the manifestations but also the mysteries of the creation.

Chapter 14: The Unfathomed Truth

Look, it is invisible.
Listen, it is inaudible.
Grab, it is intangible.

These three characteristics are indefinable:

Therefore, they are joined as one, just like the Creator—invisible, inaudible, and intangible.

As one, it is unbroken thread with neither a beginning nor an end.
It returns to nothingness: invisible, inaudible, and intangible.
It is the indefinable, the intangible, and the unimaginable.
Stand before it, and there is no beginning.
Follow it, and there is no end.
Only by its grace can we discover how things have been and will be.
This is the essence of the Creator: invisible, inaudible, and intangible.

Chapter 15: The Enlightenment

The ancient prophets were wise.
Their wisdom was unfathomable.
It is indispensable to understanding the salvation from the Creator.

All we can do is to live by their profound prophecies:
watchful, like a man crossing a winter stream;
alert, like a man aware of danger;
courteous, like a visiting guest;
yielding, like ice about to melt;
simple, like a piece of uncarved wood;
hollow, like a cave;
opaque, like muddy water.

Living by their prophecies, we wait for our muddled

thoughts to settle,
our composed minds to become clear just like
muddy water, until enlightenment arises, followed
by eternal salvation.

Chapter 16: Focusing on the Creator

Life lives itself in us, when we focus on the Creator.
From that focal point, around which all of life
revolves.

We watch everything come and go,
with no judgment, and no preference.
Everything that is, was, or ever will be,
will return to its origin: the Creator.

Understanding the comings and goings of things,
we fret not, and judge not.
Focusing on the Creator,
we are open to all of life.
Opening to all of life,
we embrace all with thankfulness for what we get,
with gratitude for not getting what we deserve.
Discovering the true nature of things,
we live with compassion and loving-kindness.
All endings become beginnings, all returning to the
Creator.

Chapter 17: No Separate Self

The greatest virtue of all is to be unaware of a
separate self at all.
Awareness of a separate self makes us want to

become valuable.

Not becoming valuable, we tend to hate the separate self.

Hating the separate self, how can we value anyone else?

Freedom from the ego-self, we are free to act without the desire to be valuable.

As a result, everything is done, and people all say: "It happened *naturally*."

Chapter 18: The Differences

In the absence of the Creator, we forget who we really are.

Then we turn to other things to define who we are, what is good and moral.

In the presence of the Creator, we act according to our hearts,

instead of relying on rules and regulations from those above us.

Rules and regulations may bring fairness and justice,

but no more than a pretense of life.

A pretense of life is our inability to love indiscriminately.

Then we insist on those above us to heal our suffering,

which originates from ourselves.

Chapter 19: Self-Intuition

Stop striving to be righteous and wise to attain salvation,
which comes not from our efforts, not something we must earn.
Stop abiding by rules and regulations to secure fairness and justice.
Compassion and loving-kindness come naturally to us.
Stop accumulating riches by being smart.
Heavenly assets are freely available to all.

The above are merely superficial suggestions.
The ultimate truths have to be self-intuited:
be simple, be selfless, and be non-judgmental.
Enlightenment may arrive effortlessly.

Chapter 20: The Creator's Wisdom

We are all desirous of making the right choices,
fearful of making the wrong ones.
We all pursue what others say is good,
avoiding what they say is bad.
We all follow the popular wisdom of judgment and preference,
instead of the wisdom of the Creator,
requiring us to be undesirous and unperturbed, just like a newborn.

The wisdom of the Creator may seem unreal, and even foolish,
while the worldly wisdom may seem smart and popular.

The Way to enlightenment and salvation is narrow and restricted,
while the way to human folly is open and wide.

The foolish all have goals.
The wise are humble and stubborn.
They alone trust the Creator,
and not the world He created.

Chapter 21: The Way

The ancient prophets follow the Way to the Creator,
the Way to re-discover our true nature,
which is being one with the Creator.

Seemingly intangible, and seemingly elusive,
the Way leads to the origin of all things,
both visible and invisible.

Since the beginning of the beginning, this has been the Way
to the life force of all things,
both past and present.

Throughout all ages, its name has been preserved.
He is the Creator of, as well as the Witness to, all existence.
Humans intuit this truth, not only by believing it, but also by living it.

Chapter 22: Everything Is Perfect

Accepting what is, we find perfection in the Creator,

as well as in everything created by Him.

What seemingly distorted is in fact truthful.
What seemingly lacking is in fact abundant.
What seemingly exhausted is in fact refreshing.

Possessing little, we become content.
Having too much, we lose the Creator.
Having no ego, we become humbled, and our actions are enlightened.
Having no desire for perfection, our actions are welcome by all.
Having no expectation of result, our actions are selfless and non-judgmental.
Having no goal, our actions are under-doing and never over-doing.

Accepting what is, and finding it to be perfect is not easy.
But that is the Way to the Creator.

Chapter 23: Nothing Lasts Forever

The Way is of few words.
Actions speak louder than words.
Strong winds come and go.
So do torrential rains.
Even heaven and earth cannot make them last forever.

Why then so much concern over what to say, or what to do?
Living is but an expression of the life given by the

Creator.
Our true nature is a reflection of that expression.
Those who are with the Creator, the Creator is also
with them.
So, success and failure are seen as part of a perfect
whole.
Everything is accepted and fully lived accordingly.

Chapter 24: Falling Short

Reaching out for it, we fall.
Running to catch it, we stumble.
Pretending to become enlightened, we become
confused.
Trying to do it right, we fail.
Looking for praise, we become disappointed.
Holding onto it, we lose.

Letting go of straining, striving, and strutting,
we find the wisdom in the Creator.

Chapter 25: The Great Mystery

The Way to the Creator existed
before the universe was created.
Its essence is formless and unchanging.
It is present wherever we turn,
providing compassion to all beings.
It comes from the Creator of the universe,
who has no name.
To identify him, just call him the Creator.
He can also be called the Great Mystery,
from whom we come, in whom we live, and to whom

we return.

The Way is great, because it is boundless.
Boundless, it is eternally flowing.
Eternally flowing, it is constantly returning.
The Way is great because it leads to our true origin,
the origin of all things in heaven and on earth.

Man follows the earth.
The earth follows the universe.
The universe follows the Creator.
The Creator follows Himself.
Hence, He is the greatest of all.

Chapter 26: Be Stable and Unmoved

The Way to the Creator is deep-rooted.
Unmoved, it is the source of all movement.
Stable, it enables us to act without rashness.

So, whatever we do, we do not abandon our true
nature.
The world around us is riddled with worries and
distractions.
We remain stable, steady, and steadfast.

We do not let ourselves be blown to and fro.
Otherwise, we lose touch with who we really are;
or, worse, who the Creator is.

Chapter 27: Pick Not, Choose Not

The Way to the Creator has no blueprint.

With faith and humility, we seek neither pride nor blame.
Our actions then become righteous and impeccable.
Our lives are illumined with the Creator's light.

Everything that happens to us is beneficial.
Everything that we experience is instructional.
Everyone that we meet, good or bad, becomes our teacher or student.

We learn from both the good and the bad.
So, stop picking and choosing.
Everything is a manifestation of the mysteries of creation.

Chapter 28: Trusting the Creator

Striving to climb the ladder of success,
we may seem smart.
But trusting our Creator,
we find divine guidance,
which is effortless along the Way.

Striving to be right or wrong according to the world,
we may seem righteous.
But trusting our Creator,
we find potentials of our true nature,
which express compassion and loving-kindness to all.

Being charismatic,
we may seem popular.
But trusting our Creator,

we find our true nature.

Separating from our true nature,
we struggle with forms and functions.
Returning to our true nature,
we find ourselves being one with the Creator.

Chapter 29: Letting Go Control

Controlling external events is futility.
Control is but an illusion.
Whenever we try to control,
we separate ourselves from our true nature.
Man proposes; the Creator disposes.
Life is sacred: it flows exactly as it should.
Trusting in the Creator, we return to our breathing,
natural and spontaneous, without conscious control.

In the same manner:
sometimes we have more,
sometimes we have less;
sometimes we exert ourselves,
sometimes we pull back;
sometimes we succeed,
sometimes we fail.

Trusting in the Creator, we see the comings and goings of things,
but without straining and striving to control them.

Chapter 30: Simplify the Doing

Letting go of control,

we no longer strive and struggle.
Without strife and struggle,
there is no resistance.
Without resistance,
there is no suffering.

Living in the present moment,
we see all things that we must do.
Without complaint and resistance, we do them
accordingly.
Without seeking control and recognition,
we simplify what we do, however complicated they
may be.
Trusting in the Creator, we always under-do and
never over-do.

Chapter 31: Forgiveness

Vengeance and violence
are not along the Way to the Creator,
no matter how justified they may be.
Faced with vengeance and violence,
remember the Creator's precepts:
forgive our enemies;
love our neighbors as ourselves.

An eye for an eye
makes us become what we hate.
Knowing this, we do not
rejoice in victory over our enemies,
nor take delight in their downfall.

Victory is but an illusion;

getting even gains us nothing.
Once vengeance and violence are over,
there is nothing left but our own pain.

Chapter 32: Beyond Words

What we call the Creator really has no name.
He is intangible and unfathomable.

We experience Him in our own true nature.
If we are one with Him, peace comes upon our lives,
like soft rain falling from heaven,
like joy rising from the earth,
like a mighty river flowing.
Our world then becomes a paradise,
and natural goodness is written in our hearts.

Since the beginning of the beginning,
there have been names for everything.
The more words we use,
the more distinctions we make.
The more distinctions we have,
the more we pick and choose.
As a result, we separate ourselves
from our own true nature.

To return to peace and harmony,
we must be like rivers and streams,
returning to their origin—the ocean.

Chapter 33: True Wisdom

Knowing others is intelligence.
Knowing ourselves is true wisdom.
Overcoming others is strength.
Overcoming ourselves is true power.

Understanding that we have everything we need,
we count our blessings.
Identifying with our own true nature,
we hold fast to what endures.

Chapter 34: Like A Great Ocean

The Creator is like an ocean.
It fills everything and everywhere.
It is the origin of life.
It never abandons its creations.
It accomplishes, but needs no recognition.
It nourishes and cherishes all,
yet gives everyone the freedom to choose.
It has no need for glory,
so it retreats to the background
and becomes inconspicuous.
Yet we all return to it.
And that is why it is great.
Its greatness needs no recognition.

Likewise, our greatness comes
not from our power or control,
but from our own true nature,
which is living as one with the Creator.

Chapter 35: Spreading the Truth

Living as one with the Creator,
there is no danger, only peace and harmony.
Lively music and gourmet food
may make people stay.
But spreading the truth about the Creator
may be unexciting and unattractive to many.
People prefer misleading distractions.
People love empty promises.

The truth about the Creator
is profound but unpopular.
Look at it; it is invisible.
Listen to it; it is inaudible.
Use it; it is inexhaustible.

Chapter 36: The Natural Laws

Before we can shrink anything,
we must first let it expand.
Before we can get rid of something,
we must first let it flourish.
Before we can receive something,
we must first give it away.
They are called the natural laws
of the way things were, are, and will be.

The soft overcomes the hard.
The slow overcomes the fast.
Gentleness and flexibility
bring positive results
that force and rigidity
fail to produce.
Just trust the natural laws

of the mighty Creator.

Chapter 37: Everything in Its Natural Place

The Creator never seems to do anything,
yet all things are done accordingly.

We stay in the very center of the Creator,
and refrain from controlling our destiny.
Everything will evolve and fall into its natural place,
according to the natural laws of the Creator.

When there is no desire to be someone that we are
not,
or to be separate from our true nature designed by
the Creator,
all things are in perfect balance and harmony.

Chapter 38: The Contrived and the Natural

The Creator has no wish to be powerful;
and thus He is truly powerful.
The ordinary man craves to be powerful;
and thus he never has enough power.

The Creator does nothing,
yet nothing is left undone.
The ordinary man is always doing things,
yet there are always many more to be done.

With the grace of the Creator,
we experience natural goodness.
Natural goodness requires no effort,

no expectation of reward or recognition.
Contrived goodness requires great effort,
with little or no accomplishment.
Compassion and loving-kindness seek nothing.
Fairness and justice demand results,
with expectation of correct behavior.
Natural goodness comes from within,
which is our essence,
and not from without,
which is only our appearance.

When we are separate from our true nature,
we experience no natural goodness,
no compassion and no loving-kindness.
Our goodness then becomes contrived,
demanding fairness and justice,
focusing on appearance and superficiality.

Chapter 39: Dependent on the Creator

Dependent on the Creator,
our horizons broaden and expand,
our souls inspire and nourish,
our relationships grow and flourish.
Everything around us becomes oneness with the Creator.

Dependent on ourselves,
our horizons contract and shrink,
our souls wither and die,
our relationships break and crumble.
Everything around us becomes depleted and damaged.

Do not strive for prestige and power.
They all belong to the Creator.
Only with humility can we connect with Him.
Humility is the Way to Him.
Dependent on the Creator,
we do not strive to be shiny like jade.
but just dull like stones.

Chapter 40: Being Born of Non-Being

Following the Way,
we return to our root.
On the Way,
yielding is the way to go.

Everything in the universe
depends on everything else.
Even living our life experience
depends on how we think of death.

Chapter 41: The Enigma

When a wise man hears of the Creator,
he immediately begins to do some soul-searching.
When an average man hears of the Creator,
he half believes Him, and half doubts Him.
When a foolish man hears of the Creator,
he laughs out loud.
If he did not laugh,
there would be no Creator.

Thus it is said:

The Way to the light seems dark.
The Way forward seems to go backward.
The Way direct seems long.
True power seems week.
True purity seems tarnished.
True steadfastness seems changeable.
True clarity seems obscure.
The greatest seems inconspicuous.
The greatest love seems indifferent.
The greatest wisdom seems foolish.

The Creator is hidden and nameless.
Yet He nourishes and completes all things.

Chapter 42: Remaining in the Center

The Creator creates one.
One creates two.
Two creates three.
Three creates a myriad of things.
All have their original unity
in the duality of the *yin* and the *yang*,
the opposite life forces that harmonize.
We experience this harmonious process
in the rising and falling of our breaths.

People naturally avoid loss and seek gain.
But with all things along the Way,
there is no need to pick and choose.
There is no gain without loss.
There is no abundance without lack.
We do not know how and when
one gives way to the other.

So, we just remain in the center of things,
trusting the Creator, instead of ourselves.
This is the essence of the Way.

Chapter 43: Effortless Effort

The softest thing in the world
overcomes what seems to be the hardest.

That which has no form
penetrates what seems to be impenetrable.

That is why we exert effortless effort.
We act without over-doing.
We teach without arguing.

This is the Way to true wisdom.
This is not a popular way
because people prefer over-doing.

Chapter 44: The Choices

Fame or self, which is dearer?
Self or wealth, which is greater?
Gain or loss, which is more painful?

Accumulating or letting go, which causes more
suffering?
Looking for status and security, we find only
suffering.
Knowing our true nature, we find joy and peace.
With nothing lacking, the whole world belongs to us.

Chapter 45: Perfectly Done

True perfection seems imperfect,
yet it is perfectly flawless.
True abundance seems lacking,
yet it is fully present.

True honesty seems hypocritical.
True wisdom seems foolish.
True eloquence seems hesitant.

When the Creator is in control,
we act with effortless effort.
What is needed is perfectly done.

Chapter 46: Lasting Satisfaction

Trusting the Creator, we concentrate on the Creator.
Relying on ourselves, we focus on our ego.

Our greatest suffering comes from
not knowing who we are, or to whom we belong.
Our greatest unhappiness comes from
wanting more than what the Creator provides.
Our greatest satisfaction of contentment
is the lasting satisfaction.

Chapter 47: Accomplish Without Striving

Without going out the door, we know the world.
Without looking out the window, we see the Creator.

The more we look outside ourselves,
the less we know about anything.

Trusting the Creator, the ancient prophets
knew without doing, understood without seeing.
Trusting the Creator, we accomplish without
striving.

Chapter 48: Need to Do Nothing

Seeking the Creator,
we give up something every day.
The less we have,
the less we need to strain and strive
until we need to do nothing.
Allowing things to come and go,
following their natural laws,
we gain everything.
Straining and striving,
we lose everything.

Chapter 49: The Creator's Mind

The Creator has no mind of His own.
He works with the mind of everyone.

He is good to those who are good.
He is also good to those who are not so good.
This is godly goodness.

He trusts those who are trustworthy.
He also trusts those who are not so trustworthy.
This is true trust.

The Creator's mind is unfathomable.
People do not understand Him.
They look up to Him and wait.
He treats them like His own children.

Chapter 50: Life and Death

Life begets death; one is inseparable from the other.
One is form; the other is formless.
Each gives way to the other.
One third of people focus on life, ignoring death.
One third of people focus on death, ignoring life.
One third of people think of neither, just drifting along.
They all suffer in the end.

Trusting the Creator, we have no illusion about life and death.
Holding nothing back from life, we are ready for death,
just as a man ready for sleep after a good day's work.

Chapter 51: In the Heart of Every Being

Each and every being in the universe
is an expression of the Creator.
We are all shaped and perfected by Him.
Therefore, we should honor the Creator
and delight in His eternal presence,
not because we are commanded,
but because it is our own nature.

The Creator gives birth to all beings,
nourishes and cherishes them,
instructs, comforts, and matures them,
and then returns them to their origin.

The Creator gives us life,
but does not claim to own us.
He is always acting on our behalf,
but expects nothing in return.
He is guiding us along the Way,
but does not control where we turn.
His presence is deep within us,
in the very nature of our being.

Chapter 52: Finding the Origin

In the beginning was the Creator.
All things originate from Him.
All things return to Him.

To find the origin,
look for His manifestations.
To find the mother,
recognize her children.
To end our suffering,
find our true nature.

Stilling our thoughts,
our needs become few.
Following our thoughts,
our distractions become more,
and thus living in chaos.

Enlightenment is our true nature.
Meditation helps us find the origin,
and thus ending our suffering.

Chapter 53: Distracting Detours

The Way is easy,
yet people prefer distracting detours.
Beware when things are out of balance.
Remain centered within the Creator.

Distractions are many,
in the form of riches and luxuries.
They allure us from the Way.
Accumulations are like extortions of the poor.
They bring only disaster and suffering.
Do not deviate from the Way.

Chapter 54: The Presence of the Creator

When we are planted in the Creator,
we will not be easily rooted up.
When we are embraced by the Creator,
we will never slip away.

If the Creator is present in our lives,
our lives will express our true nature.
If the Creator is present in our families,
our families will experience prosperity.

If the Creator is present in our countries,
our countries will set good examples

to all other countries in the world.
If the Creator is present in the universe,
the universe will delight in virtues.

How do we know this is true?
By looking inside ourselves,
when we observe the comings and goings
of everything and everyone around us.

Chapter 55: In Natural Harmony

If we are in harmony with the Creator,
we are like newborn babies,
in natural harmony with all.
Our bones are soft, and our muscles are weak,
but our grip is strong and powerful.
Not knowing about sex,
we manifest sexual arousal.
Crying all day long,
we lose not our voice.
With constancy and harmony,
we accomplish all daily tasks
without growing tired.

In natural harmony with the Creator,
we let all things come and go,
exerting no effort, showing no desire,
and expecting no result.
Natural harmony is experienced
only in the present moment,
when we see the natural laws of the Creator.

Chapter 56: No Longer Matters

The more we understand the Way,
the less we need to convince others.
Those, who speak much,
know little about the Way.

So, we no longer argue with those who are cynical.
We stop looking for their approval.
We cease taking offense at their unbelief.
We just sow the seeds along the Way,
letting the Creator reap the harvest.

To be loved or rejected,
to gain or to lose,
to be approved or disapproved,
no longer matters to us,
when we know who we are
and who the Creator is.

Chapter 57: More for Less

To guide a great country, we need a great ruler.
To wage a successful war, we need good strategies.
To live a life of harmony, we need letting life live by itself.

That essentially means:
the more efforts we exert, the more failures we experience;
the more weapons we make, the more dangers we encounter;
the more laws we enact, the more law-breakers we

produce.

So, follow the Way.
Stop striving to change ourselves: we are naturally changing.
Stop striving to be good: we are naturally good.
Stop striving to get rich: we are naturally abundant.
Stop striving to control destiny: life is naturally living itself.

Chapter 58: The Pure and Simple Way

The Way to the Creator is pure and simple.
If the Way were interfering and complicated,
it would be painful and difficult to follow.

Good fortune and misfortune are all in one.
Seeking one and rejecting the other,
we become completely confused.
Striving for goodness and righteousness,
we become evil and wicked.

To follow the Way,
we need principles,
but without imposing on others;
we need honesty,
but without being unkind to others;
we need consistency,
but without taking advantage of others.
We set an example for others
to follow the Way to the Creator.

Chapter 59: The Golden Mean

To serve others and the Creator,
there is nothing better than the golden mean.

With the golden mean, there is moderation.
With moderation, our limits are unknown.
With unknown limits, our potentials are infinite.
With infinite potentials, our power is everlasting.
With the golden mean, we accommodate ourselves to
the ever-changing world around us.
We simplify the complicated with gentle ease,
like a mother caring for her child.

Deep rooted in the presence of the golden mean,
we follow the Way, and never lose our way.

Chapter 60: Frying a Small Fish

Living our lives is like frying a small fish;
we neither over-season nor over-cook it.

Centering ourselves in the Creator,
we have neither fear nor worry.
It is not that they no longer exist,
but that they no longer have power over us.
So, they diminish and disappear from our lives.

Walking along the Way is like frying a small fish.
We used to suffer; now we have become wise.

Chapter 61: A Great Nation

A great country is like a sea,
with all streams flowing into it.
The more powerful it is,
the greater its need for humility.
Humility means trusting the Creator
in deference to the Way.

A great nation is like a great man.
When he makes a mistake,
not only does he realize it,
but also admit it.
He learns from his mistakes:
everyone is his teacher,
and his enemy is his own shadow.

If a great nation is centered in the Creator,
it cherishes and nourishes all its citizens;
it is a shining light to all other nations in the world.

Chapter 62: Abiding in the Creator

The Creator is in the center of the universe,
the refuge of those who abide in Him,
and the protector of those who ignore Him.

Honors can be bought with fine words;
respect can be won with good deeds.
Abiding in the Creator is beyond all values.

Thus, there is no greater gift of wealth and power
than showing the Way to the Creator,
just like the ancient prophets did.

Why did the ancient prophets follow the Way?
Because seeking the Creator,
we shall find what we need;
we shall find forgiveness
for the wrong we have done.
That is why everybody loves it.

Chapter 63: The Present Moment

We act without over-action.
We manage without interference.
We enjoy without attachment.

Effrontery is just
an opportunity for loving-kindness.
Great accomplishments are only
a combination of small steps.
Difficult tasks are no more than
a series of easy steps.

Therefore, we focus on the present moment,
doing what needs to be done,
without straining and stressing.

To end our suffering,
we focus on the present moment,
instead of our expected result.
So, we follow the natural laws of things.

Chapter 64: A Small Step

We need a still and composed mind
to see things with greater clarity.

Because trouble begins in the mind
with small and unrelated thoughts.
So, we carefully watch the mind
to stop any trouble before it begins.
Thus we put things in order
before they become out of order.

The great pine tree
springs from a tiny sprout.
The journey of a thousand miles
begins with the first step.

Accordingly, we do not rush into things.
We neither strain nor stress.
We let go of success and failure.
We patiently take the next necessary step,
a small step and one step at a time.
We relinquish our conditioned thinking.
Being our true nature, we help all beings
return to their own true nature too.

Chapter 65: Humble Simplicity

The ancient prophets used simple ways
to teach the Way to the Creator.

Those, who think they know, know not the Way.
Those, who think they know not, find the Way.

Simplicity is clarity.
It is a blessing to learn from those
with humble simplicity.
Those with an empty mind

will learn to find the Way.
The Way reveals the secrets of the universe:
the mysteries of the realm of creation;
the manifestations of all things created.
The essence of the Way is to show us
how to live in fullness and return to our origin.

Chapter 66: The Power of Humility

Rivers and streams generate great power
as they flow down to the ocean below.
The power is in the downward movement

Humility is power.
Power comes from the lowly.
According to the Way:
the lowly will be elevated;
the last will be the first.

The Creator is above,
and we are below.
The Creator is in front,
and we are behind.
Because this is the nature of things,
humility is only natural to us.
Yet many are desirous of the top
fearful of lagging behind.
Humility is the Way.

Chapter 67: The Three Essentials

The Way may seem insignificant.
It is because it appears ordinary.

The Way is great beyond comparison.
If there were any comparison,
it would no longer be great.

The Way is great because of its three essentials:
compassion, humility, and faith.
With compassion, there is no fear.
With humility, there is no strife.
With faith, there is no impossibility.

Without compassion, fearlessness becomes
ruthlessness.
Without humility, efforts become complicated and
difficult.
Without faith, possibilities become controlling and
self-centering.

Compassion is the root.
Humility is the stem.
Faith is the flower.

Chapter 68: Not Seeking Our Way

We do not become aggressive when we are
confronted.
We do not become angry when we are provoked.
We see neither an enemy nor a competitor,
because we do not seek our own way.

Knowing both our strengths and weaknesses,
we use them to complement one another.
Thus, we find balance and harmony.
Naturally and easily, we follow the Way.

Chapter 69: Become Our Own Enemy

According to military strategies,
defense is preferred to attack;
consolidation is better than overextension.

So, we advance
not at the expense of overstepping anyone.
So, we gain
not at the expense of making anyone lose.
So, we accomplish
not at the expense of straining ourselves.

We have no enemy.
We love everyone as ourselves.
We remain in our true nature;
otherwise, we lose
the three essentials of the Way,
and become our own enemy.

Chapter 70: Easy to Find and Follow

The Way is easy to find and follow:
empty the mind of conditioned thinking
of seeing things and doing things.

The Way comes from the source of all.
Its power cherishes and nourishes all.
Knowing the source, we know ourselves.

Finding the Way,
we know the nature of things;

we see the comings and goings of things.

Following the Way,
we discover the treasures within;
we simplify the trappings without.
So, we continue the Way with inner joy.

Chapter 71: The Importance of Knowing

Not knowing the Way,
but pretending we know,
we remain ignorant, and suffer.

Knowing that we do not know,
we pursue its wisdom:
knowing its origin,
knowing its ending,
and knowing our true nature.

Chapter 72: In Awe of the Creator

Without awe of the mysteries of the Creator,
we are easily controlled by fear.
Without self-love and compassion for others,
we are easily victimized by others.

Knowing our true nature,
we know who we are,
and what we need.
We accomplish things
without taking credit or reward.
We cherish ourselves
without separating us from other beings.

We nourish our external identity
without forgetting our inner reality.

Chapter 73: Nothing Slips Through

We try to be good, and do the best we can,
yet sometimes bad things happen to us.
We have no explanation for that.
We just follow the Way,
one step at a time,
accepting the good and the bad,
as essential parts of life.
We quietly respond to every situation
with neither strain nor stress.

We trust the Creator.
His net, vast and loose,
covers the whole universe,
and nothing slips through.
He controls all.

Chapter 74: Unnatural Fear of Death

Abiding in the Creator, we do not fear death.
Following the conditioned mind, we fear everything.
Fear is a futile attempt to control things and people.

Death is a natural destination of the Way.
Unnatural fear of death does more harm than good.
It is like trying to use intricate tools of a master
craftsman:
we end up hurting ourselves.

Chapter 75: Never Really Live

When there is abundance, there is lacking.
When there is craving, there is discontentment.
Striving for power to control and influence
every aspect of our lives
is the source of our suffering.

Obsessed with getting and keeping,
many of us never really live before we die.

Following the Way,
we must learn to let go.

Chapter 76: Soft and Yielding

At birth, we are soft and supple.
At death, we are stiff and hard.
Young plants are tender and pliant.
Dead plants are brittle and dry.

Stiff and inflexible, we are like death.
Soft and yielding, we are like life.

Following the Way,
we become soft and supple.
That is why we always prevail,
because tenderness and flexibility
give us strength and power from the Creator.

Chapter 77: Like Bending a Bow

Following the Way is like bending a bow:

one end is pulled up;
the other end is pulled down.
Excess and deficiency are balanced.

According to the wisdom of the Way:
we reduce when there is excess;
we increase when there is deficiency.
Balance is thus created.

According to common wisdom:
we increase excess and deplete deficiency.
Imbalance is thus created.

Following the Way,
we follow our true nature:
giving without worrying;
receiving without attaching.

Chapter 78: The Paradox

The Way is paradoxical.
Like water, soft and yielding,
yet it overcomes the hard and the rigid.
Stiffness and stubbornness cause much suffering.

We all intuitively know
that flexibility and tenderness
are the Way to go.
Yet our conditioned mind
tells us to go the other way.

We accept all that is simple and humble.
We embrace the good fortune and the misfortune.

Thus, we become masters of every situation.
We overcome the painful and the difficult in our lives.
That is why the Way seems paradoxical.

Chapter 79: True Contentment

Resentment breeds more resentment.
Only contentment leads to contentment.
True contentment comes from our true nature:
not from what we do, or how we do;
neither from our status nor our control.

The Creator is impartial.
No one is special.

Chapter 80: Feeling Contented

Living in the present moment,
we find natural contentment.
We do not seek a faster lifestyle,
or a better place to be.
We need the essentials of life,
not its extra trimmings.

Living in the present moment,
we focus on the experience of the moment.
Thus, we enjoy every aspect of simple living,
and find contentment in everyone and everything.

Living in contentment,
we grow old and die,
feeling contented.

Chapter 81: True Wisdom

The truth is unpleasant to the ear.
What is pleasant to the ear is not the truth.
Likewise, true wisdom is unpopular;
what is popular is not true wisdom.

The wise learn to let go, instead of accumulating.
The wise learn to succumb, instead of arguing.
The wise find the Way, not from knowledge,
but from their own true nature.

Without straining and striving for control,
we discover what life really is:
following the Way to the Creator.

The TAO Essentials

Despite its apparent mysticism and paradoxical nature, TAO or "the Way" is not difficult to understand. All you need is an empty mind with *reverse* thinking from the conventional way of conditioned thinking.

There was the well-known story of a professor visiting a Zen master and seeking information about Zen (an ancient Asian philosophy evolved from the TAO). The Zen master kept pouring tea into the already filled-up teacup in the professor's hand, while the professor continued his talking. The moral of the story: you must keep an empty mind before you can be open and receptive to any new idea;

having a pre-conditioned mindset is a common characteristic of the contemporary human mind.

According to Lao Tzu, the essentials of TAO cannot be expressed in words. As a matter of fact, words in themselves are not important because they are not the truths. They do not teach; they only *point* to the truths. There is a saying: "The teacher and the taught together create the teaching." Teaching is the embodiment of *awareness*, *assimilation*, and *application* of understanding, without which there is no learning or teaching, not to mention true wisdom. In other words, the TAO is all about your own *understanding*: of the self, of others, as well as of things around the self. But nobody can *make* you understand—not even words—and only your own *thinking mind* can.

Humility

If the TAO could be expressed in one word, maybe that one word would be "humility."

What is meant by "humility" according to Lao Tzu?

Humility has to do with the *self*, which has to do with the mind, which has to do with the thinking process, and which has to do with human thoughts. They all have to do with the *ego-self*.

No Fear, No Expectation

Human fear comes in different forms: instinctive

fear, such as fear of a dangerous environment; and psychological fear, such as anxiety, paranoia, and worry. The former is more natural and grounded than the latter, which is based more on the factor "might." But all fear has to do with failure and ultimately death. Once you have illusively identified yourself with that fear in your mind, the fear begins to overtake you as a person and you then become the very thing you are afraid of.

Consumed with fear, your mind then begins to expect something different from what you fear. But with no fear, there is no expectation.

No Judgment, No Pain

Human life is never pain-free or sorrow-free. Failures and frustrations—they all come from expectations—often lead to human pain and stress.

Fear of human pain further intensifies your mind to pick and choose: picking what you think will help you avoid the imaginary pain; and choosing what you think will help you fulfill your expectation. In the process of choosing and judging, you often make mistakes and wrong choices, and thus creating only more fear and more pain, as well as leading to vicious circles of expectations and frustrations.

Natural Cycles

According to the TAO, these extremes in human experiences are not only temporary but also unnatural; they are just the cycles of nature in which the pendulum swings back and forth from one end to the other.

It is human folly to attempt to avoid or resist experiencing these swings; by doing so, man throws himself out of balance with nature, and thus not only intensifies but also unduly prolongs his pain and suffering.

No Over-Doing

The TAO emphasizes "wu-wei" (無為): "Wu" (無) means "no" and "wei" (為) means "doing." Due to the literal translation of the original text, "wu-wei" is often misinterpreted as "non-doing," and therefore even regarded as a "passive" way of looking at life by Lao Tzu. "Under-doing" or "nothingness" is a more appropriate translation of "wu-wei."

Living in the Present

According to the TAO, only the present is real: the past was already gone, and the future, uncertain and unpredictable, is yet to come. When the mind stays in the present, it has clarity of thinking that does not see the ego-self. But when the mind constantly alternates between the past and the future, it then becomes self-deceptive and self-delusional, and thus creating the false ego-self.

Letting Go

Living in the present enables clarity of mind, and hence the capability of the mind to let go of everything, including the ego. With no ego, there is no expectation; with no expectation, there is no picking and choosing; with no picking and choosing, there is no fear and disappointment, and hence no stress.

FOUR

NO EGO NO STRESS

Understanding the TAO is not that difficult, or is it? Practicing the TAO to cope with your everyday life stressors may be more challenging, especially if you do not have an empty mind with reverse thinking.

"Accepting what is, and finding it to be perfect
is not easy.
But that is the only Way to the Creator."
(Chapter 22, *Tao Te Ching*)

There are five major life stressors: career, money, relationship, adversity, and time. They have become part and parcel of life that they are now the norm.

But with no ego, there is no stress in the first place.

Career Stress

Career is a major stressor in contemporary living: one of the obvious reasons is that it normally spans over several decades of a person's life, involving many changes and challenges, as well as many ups and downs.

With no ego, you choose a career that goes with your life passion, rather than one just to satisfy your own desire for recognition and remuneration, or simply to defer to the wish of someone else, such as your parents. That is to say, do what you like, and like what you do. If you wish to be an artist, then seek your career as one, even though your parents may want you to become a doctor or a lawyer.

"Fame or self, which is dearer?
The self or wealth, which is greater?
Gain or loss, which is more painful?
(Chapter 44, *Tao Te Ching*)

A case in point is that many students in a community college choose nursing as their career simply because they think they will be able to find a job in the medical field when they graduate. But do they *really* want to serve patients in a hospital setting? If they do not, then going to work every day will not be a pleasant and rewarding experience. Also, do they have a basic math background? If they do not, then struggling in a math class in a community college is a stressful experience itself.

The bottom line: with no ego, there is no stress in your career choice.

"We are all desirous of making the right choices,
fearful of making the wrong ones.
We all pursue what others say is good,
Avoiding what they say is bad.
We all follow the popular wisdom of judgment and preference,

Instead of the wisdom of the Creator."
(Chapter 20, *Tao Te Ching*)

With no ego, you are more in harmony with your co-workers, clients or customers. Having an ego is an intense experience of "me": according to **Albert Einstein**, it is a sense of being "separate" from the rest of the universe, and is therefore an "optical delusion of consciousness."

> "The greatest virtue of all is to be unaware of a separate self at all.
> Awareness of a separate self makes us want to become valuable.
> Not becoming valuable, we tend to hate the separate self.
> Hating the separate self, how can we value anyone else?
>
> Freedom from the ego-self, we are free to act without the desire to be valuable.
> As a result, everything is done, and people all say: "It happened *naturally*."
> (Chapter 17, *Tao Te Ching*)

Having no separate self is a reflection of your interconnection with others that often leads to better relationships with those you encounter along your career pathways. Having better relationships with others means having less or no stress.

The bottom line: with no ego, you see others as yourself, and therefore they do not stress you.

With no ego, you do not feel that you are not good enough for the job. With that negative self-belief, you often send that same message to others as well, and they, too, will think that you are not good enough; and thus attracting and creating everything negative that happens to you in your work.

The bottom line: with no ego, you see yourself neither competent nor incompetent—you are just *you* doing your best in your work.

"Living in the present moment,
we see all things that we must do.
Without complaint and resistance, we do them accordingly.
Without seeking control and recognition,
we simplify what we do, however complicated they may be.
Trusting in the Creator, we always under-do and never over-do."
(Chapter 30, *Tao Te Ching*)

With no ego, you do not have to comply with the unrealistic demands of employers or coworkers, and you do not have to argue with them over this and that, or rules and regulations.

"Rules and regulations may bring fairness and justice,
but no more than a pretense of life.
A pretense of life is our inability to love indiscriminately.

Then we insist on those above us to heal our suffering,
which originates from ourselves."
(Chapter 18, *Tao Te Ching*"

"To follow the Way,
we need principles,
but without imposing on others;
we need honesty,
but without being unkind to others;
we need consistency,
but without taking advantage of others.
We set an example for others
to follow the Way to the Creator."
(Chapter 58, *Tao Te Ching*)

The bottom line: with no ego, you do what needs to be done without the stress of over-doing or doing more to guarantee your success.

With no ego, you do not have to overwork yourself in order to prove your invaluable contributions or indispensable role.

"The softest thing in the world
overcomes what seems to be the hardest.

That which has no form
penetrates what seems to be impenetrable.

That is why we exert effortless effort.
We act without over-doing.
We teach without arguing.

This is the Way to true wisdom.
This is not a popular way
because people prefer over-doing."
(Chapter 43, *Tao Te Ching*)

There was a Chinese story . . . (畫蛇添足) about a drawing competition, in which candidates were asked to draw a snake in detail. One of the candidates finished his drawing sooner than all the rest of the competitors. Thinking that extra effort might give him extra credit, he took it upon himself to add to the snake some legs with fine details. As a result of his extra effort, instead of "non-doing," he was disqualified and lost the competition.

With no ego, you do not have to control or manipulate others in order to have a successful career.

"Letting go control,
we no longer strive and struggle.
Without strife and struggle,
there is no resistance.
Without resistance,
there is no suffering."
(Chapter 30, *Tao Te Ching*)

With no ego, you do not have to push over others while climbing your own career ladder, and you do not become disappointed when someone has overtaken you in your career advancement.

With no ego, you do not worry about your job security. After all, worrying is no more than the expectation of "what if" or "what might."

> "So, whatever we do, we do not abandon our true nature.
> The world around us is riddled with worries and distractions.
> We remain stable, steady, and steadfast."
> (Chapter 26, *Tao Te Ching*)

With no ego, unemployment is only a natural cycle to generate yet another job opportunity for you. .

No ego, no career stress.

Money Stress

Money is another major stressor, whether you have too little or too much money.

With no ego, you do not have to keep up with the Joneses.

> "Accumulating or letting go, which causes more suffering?
> Looking for status and security, we find only suffering.
> Knowing our true nature, we find joy and peace.
> With nothing lacking, the whole world belongs to us."
> (Chapter 44, *Tao Te Ching*)

With no ego, you do not buy things you do not need with the money you do not have.

"Understanding that we have everything we need,
we count our blessings.
Identifying with our true nature,
we hold fast to what endures."
(Chapter 33, *Tao Te Ching*)

With no ego, you lead a simple life, instead of a luxurious one.

"Just be simple, be selfless, and be non-judgmental.
Enlightenment may arrive effortlessly."
(Chapter 19, *Tao Te Ching*)

"Living by the Spirit, we choose a simple and humble lifestyle.
We meditate to enhance our spirituality.
We love our neighbors as ourselves.
We express compassion to all.
We speak with truth and sincerity.
We live in the present moment.
We take action only when necessary.

Without much ado or over-doing, we trust the guidance of the Spirit.
In this manner, life flows like water, fulfilling itself and also everything naturally."
(Chapter 8, *Tao Te Ching*)

With no ego, you do not worry about living from hand to mouth, or what you are going to do with your money, just as **Robert Kennedy** once said: "Sometimes I think that the only people in this country who worry more about money than the poor are the very wealthy. They worry about losing it, they worry about how it is invested, they worry about the effect it's going to have. And as the zeroes increase, the dilemmas get bigger." Having little or lots of money makes little difference in living a simple lifestyle. Stress comes from wanting more and more.

"In the same manner:
sometimes we have more,
sometimes we have less;
sometimes we exert ourselves,
sometimes we pull back;
sometimes we succeed,
sometimes we fail."
(Chapter 29, *Tao Te Ching*)

With no ego, you understand the futility of using money to control others.

"Controlling external events is futility.
Control is but an illusion.
Whenever we try to control,
we separate ourselves from our true nature.
Man proposes; the Creator disposes."
(Chapter 29, *Tao Te Ching*)

"Likewise, our greatness comes
not from our power or control,
but from our own true nature,
which is living as one with the Creator."
(Chapter 34, *Tao Te Ching*)

With no ego, you realize that you cannot take it with
you when you leave this world.

"We watch everything come and go,
with no judgment, no preference.
Everything that is, was, or ever will be,
will return to its origin: the Creator."
(Chapter 16, *Tao Te Ching*)

No ego, no money stress.

Relationship Stress

John Donne, the famous poet, says: "No man is an
island" That is to say, we are all interconnected with
one another, either directly or indirectly. With ego,
this intricate interconnection may result in daily
stress in the form of conflicts and arguments:
stressful relationships between couples, between
friends, between parents and children, between
grandchildren and grandparents. Relationship is
always a major stressor in life.

With ego, you see yourself as "special" and "not just
like others."

With ego, you see imperfections in others, but not in

yourself. Accordingly, you expect others to satisfy your ego; and if they fall short of that, disharmony and dissatisfaction occur, resulting in conflicts and arguments.

With no ego, you see yourself as others, with no judgment of self and others, and hence no aggression and no expectation.

"We do not become aggressive when we are confronted.
We do not become angry when we are provoked.
We see neither an enemy nor a competitor, because we do not seek our own way.

Knowing both our strengths and weaknesses, we use them to complement one another.
Thus, we find balance and harmony.
Naturally and easily, we follow the Way."
(Chapter 68, *Tao Te Ching*)

With no ego, you understand the positive significance of "no man is an island": you are not much different from others around you—they all need love and compassion, just as you do.

"To be loved or rejected,
to gain or to lose,
to be approved or disapproved,
no longer matters to us,
when we know who we are
and who the Creator is."

(Chapter 56, *Tao Te Ching*)

With no ego, you discover your own innate natural goodness, just as you see the goodness in others.

"Natural goodness requires no effort,
no expectation of reward or recognition.
Contrived goodness requires great effort,
with little or no accomplishment.
Compassion and loving-kindness seek nothing.
Fairness and justice demand results,
with expectation of correct behavior.
Natural goodness comes from within,
which is our essence,
and not from without,
which is only our appearance."
(Chapter 38, *Tao Te Ching*)

With ego, you experience only contrived and superficial goodness, always demanding fairness and justice from others.

With no ego, you learn compliance rather than defiance, tolerance rather than having your way or no way.

"The soft overcomes the hard.
The slow overcomes the fast.
Gentleness and flexibility
bring positive results
that force and rigidity
fail to produce.
Just trust the natural laws

of the mighty Creator."
(Chapter 36, *Tao Te Ching*)

With no ego, there is no need to strive to change your true self, or to change others to meet your expectations.

"Stop striving to change ourselves: we are naturally changing.
Stop striving to be good: we are naturally good.
Stop striving to get rich: we are naturally abundant.
Stop striving to control destiny: life is naturally living itself."
(Chapter 57, *Tao Te Ching*)

With no ego, there is always appreciation, contentment, and gratification.

"Resentment breeds more resentment.
Only contentment leads to contentment.
True contentment comes from our true nature:
not from what we do, or how we do;
neither from our status nor our control."
(Chapter 79, *Tao Te Ching*)

"An eye for an eye
makes us become what we hate.
Knowing this, we do not
rejoice in victory over our enemies,
nor take delight in their downfall.

Victory is but an illusion;
getting even gains us nothing.
Once vengeance and violence are over,
there is nothing left but our own pain.
(Chapter 31, *Tao Te Ching*)

With no ego, there is always room and readiness for compassion, confidence, and trust toward others.

The Way is great because of its three essentials:
compassion, humility, and faith.
With compassion, there is no fear.
With humility, there is no strife.
With faith, there is no impossibility.

Without compassion, fearlessness becomes ruthlessness.
Without humility, efforts become complicated and difficult.
Without faith, possibilities become controlling and self-centering.

Compassion is the root.
Humility is the stem.
Faith is the flower.
(Chapter 67, *Tao Te Ching*)

No ego, no relationship stress.

Adversity Stress

As life continues, adversity and loss may come in

many different forms, such as loss of health, loss of mobility, and loss of loved ones, among others. Death and bereavement are inevitable human tragedies. They are some of the life challenges and adversities that we must all confront sooner or later.

"Can we embrace both good fortunes and misfortunes in life?
Can we breathe as easily as innocent babies?
Can we see the world created as is without judgment?
Can we accept both the desirable and the undesirable?
Can we express compassion to all without being boastful?
Can we watch the comings and goings of things without being perturbed?"
(Chapter 10, *Tao Te Ching*)

With no ego, there is no success or failure, no happiness or unhappiness, only acceptance and embracing.

"Success and failure are no more than expressions of the human condition.
So, accept both gracefully and willingly, with no judgment, no preference.
The Creator loves us unconditionally, irrespective of our success or failure.
What is meant by "accept both gracefully and willingly"?
Success is avoiding failure; avoiding failure is seeking success.

Both originate from fear and pride: the sources
of human suffering."
(Chapter 13, **Lao Te Ching**)

With no ego, you become enlightened: that good
fortune and misfortune are all in one, that all things
follow a natural cycle, just like the four seasons, and
that your greatest unhappiness stems from your
wanting good things to last indefinitely, instead of
allowing them to come and go, following their own
natural cycles.

"People naturally avoid loss and seek gain.
But with all things along the Way,
there is no need to pick and choose.
There is no gain without loss.
There is no abundance without lack.
We do not know how and when
one gives way to the other."
(Chapter 42, **Tao Te Ching**)

With no ego, there is no adversity, only an
opportunity for another life transformation.

"Understanding the comings and goings of
things,
we fret not, and judge not.
Focusing on the Creator,
we are open to all of life.
Opening to all of life,
we embrace all with thankfulness for what we
get,
with gratitude for not getting what we deserve.

Discovering the true nature of things,
we live with compassion and loving-kindness.
All endings become beginnings, all returning
to the Creator."
(Chapter 16, *Tao Te Ching*)

There was a Chinese story . . . 塞翁失馬 about a man who lost his only horse, which ran away one day. His friends comforted him. But he was not upset; instead, he said: "That's not a misfortune." A few days later, his horse came back with a stallion. This time, his friends congratulated him on his good fortune. But he said: "What's so good about that?" Later on, his son rode on the stallion and accidentally broke his leg when he fell from the stallion. Once again, his friends comforted him. But he said: "Breaking his leg may not be a misfortune." Indeed, soon after that, a war broke out, and all the young men in the community were drafted into the army, except the man's son with a broken leg. All of them were later annihilated in a fierce battle. The moral of the story: a misfortune may turn itself into a good fortune.

"Everything that happens to us is beneficial.
Everything that we experience is instructional.
Everyone that we meet, good or bad, becomes our teacher or student.

We learn from both the good and the bad.
So, stop picking and choosing.
Everything is a manifestation of the mysteries of creation."

(Chapter 27, *Tao Te Ching*)

With no ego, you embrace death and bereavement with peace of mind.

"Life begets death; one is inseparable from the other.
One is form; the other is formless.
Each gives way to the other.
One third of people focus on life, ignoring death.
One third of people focus on death, ignoring life.
One third of people think of neither, just drifting along.
They all suffer in the end."
(Chapter 50, *Tao Te Ching*)

No ego, no adversity stress.

Time Stress

You are living in a compulsive world, and time is always compressive and stressful.

"In natural harmony with the Creator,
we let all things come and go,
exerting no effort, showing no desire,
and expecting no result.
Natural harmony is experienced
only in the present moment,
when we see the natural laws of the Creator."
(Chapter 55, *Tao Te Ching*)

With no ego, there is no need of over-doing, which

often creates time stress in the process.

"Therefore, we focus on the present moment,
doing what needs to be done,
without straining and stressing.

To end our suffering,
we focus on the present moment,
instead of our expected result.
So, we follow the natural laws of things."
(Chapter 63, *Tao Te Ching*)

With no ego, there is no need of going back to the past, or looking forward to the future. With no ego, you simply live in the present.

"Living in the present moment,
we find natural contentment.

We do not seek a faster lifestyle,
or a better place to be.
We need the essentials of life,
not its extra trimmings.

Living in the present moment,
we focus on the experience of the moment.
Thus, we enjoy every aspect of simple living,
and find contentment in everyone and
everything."
(Chapter 81, *Tao Te Ching*)

No ego, no time stress.

Final Words of Wisdom

There are many conventional ways to cope with stress. But the most effective way comes from within, and not from without; after all, stress comes from the self, and therefore the most logical solution should also derive from the self. That is to say, stress originates from the ego-self, and therefore letting go of the ego is the perfect and the ultimate solution.

To let go of the ego, you need to know who you are, and not what you *think* you are or wish you were.

"Knowing our true nature,
we know who we are,
and what we need.
We accomplish things
without taking credit or reward.
We cherish ourselves
without separating us from other beings.
We nourish our external identity
without forgetting our inner reality."
(Chapter 72, *Tao Te Ching*)

Knowing your true nature through awareness and clarity of mind is the beginning of wisdom, which has little to do with knowledge, but much to do with your perception and your processing of all your life experiences.

"Not knowing the Way,
but pretending we know,

we remain ignorant, and suffer.

Knowing that we do not know,
we pursue its wisdom:
knowing its origin,
knowing its ending,
and knowing our true nature."
(Chapter 71, *Tao Te Ching*)

Wisdom is essentially understanding of the true nature of *all* things—the mysteries of the realm of creation and the manifestations of all things created.

"When there is no desire to be someone that we are not,
separate from our true nature designed by the Creator,
all things are in perfect balance and harmony."
(Chapter 37, *Tao Te Ching*)

"The essence of the Way is to show us
how to live in fullness and return to our origin."
(Chapter 65, *Tao Te Ching*"

Attaining this profound human wisdom is self-enlightenment, which requires an empty mind with revere thinking.

"An empty mind with no craving and no expectation helps us let go of everything.
Being in the world and not of the world, we attain heavenly grace.

With heavenly grace, we become pure and selfless.
And everything settles into its own perfect place."
(Chapter 3, *Tao Te Ching*)

Self-enlightenment is letting go of everything, including the ego. With no ego, you see the world in a different or *reverse* way—just like a person, who was born blind, suddenly opens his eyes and sees the world for the first time. With self-enlightenment, you become a different person, and the world looks totally different too.

Stephen Lau

ABOUT THE AUTHOR

About the Author
http://www.stephencmlau.com

Books by the Author:
http://www.booksbystephenlau.com

Contact Stephen Lau
stephencmlau@gmail.com